A MUST READ FOR ACUPUNCTURISTS, HERBALISTS, NATUROPATHS, MEDICAL DOCTORS, AND FUNCTIONAL MEDICINE PRACTITIONERS

Functional Herbal Medicine and Phytonutrition

A Timely Review of Astragalus Polysaccharides, Glycyrrhizin, Baicalin, Scutellarein, Amygdalin, Atractylon, Kaempferol, Luteolin, Quercetin, Emodin, Artemisinin, Forsythoside A, Saikosaponin B2, Platycodon D, Allicin, Gingerols, Cinnamaldehyde, Chlorogenic Acid, and Ginsenosides for Viral Respiratory Infections

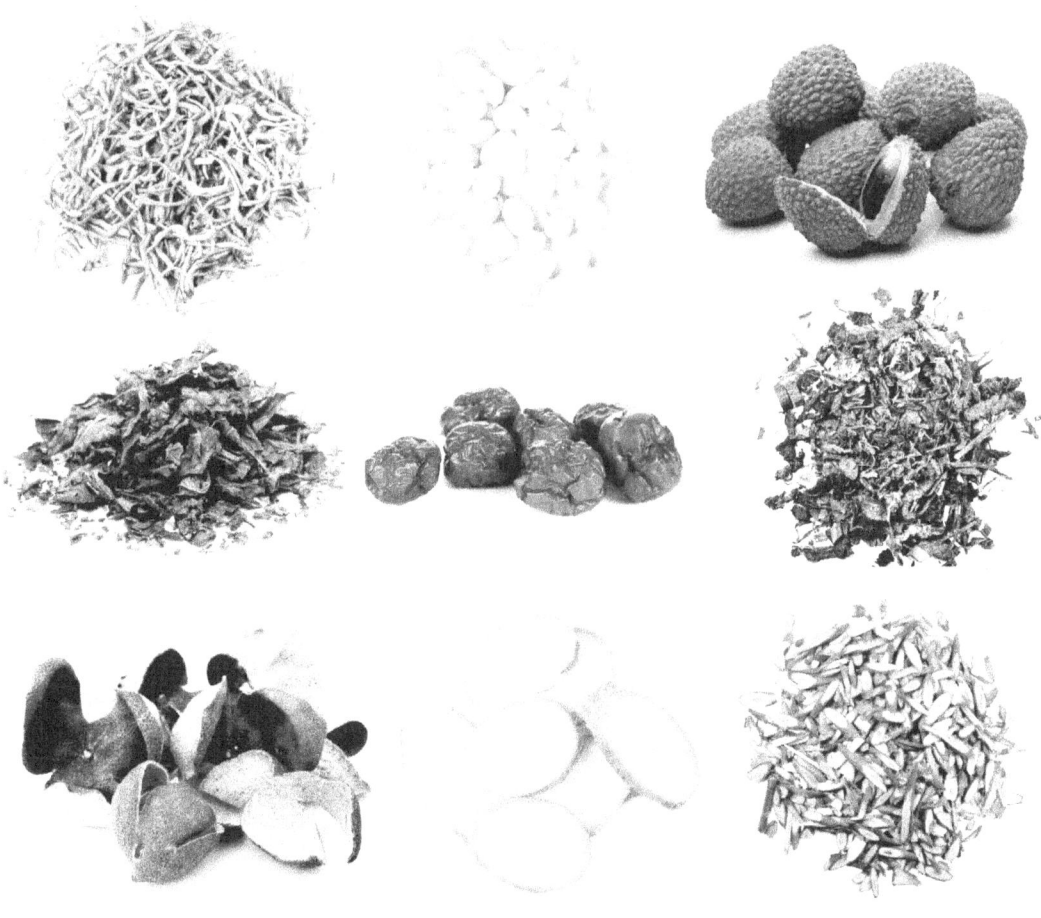

ANNE ANGELONE, MSTCM, DACM, L.AC.

Copyright © by Anne Angelone, 2020

All Rights Reserved

ISBN: 9798654287878

No part of this publication may be reproduced in any form or by any means, including scanning, photocopying, or otherwise without prior written permission of the copyright holder. Image credits: with permission from dreamstime.com

Disclaimer: This text is not intended to provide medical advice or to take the place of medical advice and treatment from your physician. The information in this text has not been evaluated by the U.S. Food and Drug Administration. Readers are advised to consult their doctors or other qualified health professionals regarding the treatment of medical conditions.

The author shall not be held liable or responsible for any misunderstanding or misuse of the information contained in this manual or for any loss, damage, or injury caused or alleged to be caused directly or indirectly by any treatment, action, or application of the nutritional model discussed in this text. This information is not intended to diagnose, treat, cure, or prevent any disease. To request permission for reproduction, please contact:

Website: www.anneangelone.com

Table of Contents

PART I Potent Plant Compounds 5

   Introduction 5

   Antiviral Compounds..6

   Important Polyphenols and Phytochemicals..8

   Functional Flavonoids..9

   Herbs for Viral Respiratory Infections...14

   SARS-CoV-2 Genomics, Transmission, and Risk Factors 16

   Viral Targets for SARS-CoV-2 Inhibition 17

   ACE2 Blockade..18

   $3CL^{pro}/M^{pro}$ Inhibition *24*

   PL^{pro} Inhibition *32*

   Spike Protein Binding..34

   Helicase Inhibition 35

   RNA-dependent RNA polymerase (RdRp) Inhibition.......................38

   Viroporin 3a Ion Channel Inhibition 39

   TMPRSS2 Inhibition..39

   The Synergistic Effect..39

PART II Review of Herbal Formulas for Viral Respiratory Infections..**42**

   Herbal Medicine for Viral Epidemics..43

   Yu Ping Feng San – Jade Screen Powder *45*

   Sang Ju Yin – Mulberry Leaf and Chrysanthemum Decoction..... *48*

   Ge Gen Tang – Kudzu Decoction *56*

   Chai Ge Jie Ji Tang – Bupleurum and Pueraria Combination *60*

   Huo Xiang Zheng Qi Wan – Agastache Formula to Rectify the Qi............... *64*

Yin Qiao San – Honeysuckle and Forsythia Powder 70

Lian Hua Qing Wen Capsule 77

Shuang Huang Lian 85

Bai Hu Tang – White Tiger Decoction 90

Qing Fei Pai Du Tang – Clear the Lung and Eliminate Toxins Decoction 91

Ma Xing Shi Gan Tang – Decoction of Ephedra, Apricot Kernel, Gypsum, and Licorice 106

Xiao Chai Hu Tang – Minor Bupleurum Decoction 107

She Gan Ma Huang Tang – Belamcanda and Ephedra Decoction 107

Wu Ling San – Five-Ingredient Powder with Poria 109

Qing Qi Hua Tan Wan – Clear the Qi and Transform Phlegm Pill 110

Ding Chuan Tang – Arrest Wheezing Decoction 110

Sheng Mai San – Generate the Pulse Powder 118

Sha Shen Mai Dong Tang – Glehnia and Ophiopogonis Decoction 120

Safety of Medicinal Herbs 122

PART III The Role of Phytochemistry and Nutrition 124

Nutrigenomics - Modulating NFKB and Cytokines 124

Common NFKB Inhibitors 126

The Gut-Lung Axis and Phytonutrient Dense Foods 127

Glutathione, N-acetyl-cysteine, and Alpha-Lipoic Acid 134

Mannose-Binding Lectins 135

Final Thoughts 136

About Anne Angelone, MSTCM, DACM, L.AC. 138

References 140

More books by Anne Angelone 176

PART I

Potent Plant Compounds

INTRODUCTION

People have been seeking traditional herbal medicines for various viral respiratory disorders, including the common cold, influenza, bronchitis, and pneumonia for hundreds of years. However, the bioactive ingredients in traditional herbs have only recently come to light in the past few decades. In Functional Herbal Medicine and Phyronutrition, we will investigate the synergistic use of potent plant compounds in common foods, traditional herbs, and formulas for viral respiratory infections. We will also review virtual screening and molecular docking analyses of individual herbs, network pharmacology analyses of herbal formulas, and clinical studies that shine a new light on potent compounds in traditional herbs and their actions.

Some of the most effective compounds, including glycyrrhizin, baicalin, scutellarin, kaempferol, luteolin, quercetin, emodin, amygdalin, forsythoside A, saikosaponin B2, platycodin D, ginsenosides, lonicerin, and chlorogenic acid, will be explored. Combining these compounds in herbal formulas provides a three-hit antiviral, immune-modulating, and anti-inflammatory effect to help decrease the severity of infections, modulate immune activity, and reduce inflammation.

One purpose of this book is to encourage practitioners to learn to identify the potent plant constituents found in traditional formulas for viral respiratory infections that make them so useful. For example, flavonoids such as the flavone luteolin, and the flavonols kaempferol and quercetin, are ubiquitous in Chinese herbs used for viral respiratory infections. Another purpose of this book is to encourage practitioners to identify the common foods that contain these same compounds. As you will discover, kaempferol, luteolin, quercetin, and other potent polyphenols in everyday fruits and vegetables, can be included in the diet to add to the synergistic effects of traditional herbs. This herbal and dietary approach has been used for centuries yet has only recently been described in phytochemical and epigenetic terms that may even surprise many acupuncturists. With this understanding, let's begin with a review of antiviral compounds contained in routinely used herbs that have synergistic effects in multi-herb formulas.

ANTIVIRAL COMPOUNDS

Traditional medicines have been used for viral infections and many other disorders that involve immune activity and inflammation for centuries. Many herbs used in Traditional Chinese Medicine (TCM) have demonstrated antiviral effects (Wang et al., 2014; Schwarz et al., 2014; Cinatl et al., 2003). Importantly, an increasing amount of current research confirms that flavonoids in Chinese herbs such as kaempferol, luteolin, quercetin, and baicalin may be useful for blocking viral entry, and inhibiting viral replication of SARS-CoV-2 (Zhang et al., 2020; Chen & Du, 2020; Niu et al., 2020).

The antiviral compounds in the herbs and formulas that we will review are comprised of various types of phytochemicals, including, but not limited to alkaloids (e.g., berberine), phenolic compounds, such as flavonoids (e.g., baicalin, quercetin, kaempferol, luteolin, and apigenin), phenylpropanoids (e.g., chlorogenic acid), terpenoids (e.g., glycyrrhizin), anthraquinones (e.g., emodin), polysaccharides (e.g., astragalus polysaccharides), saikosaponins (e.g., saiksaponin B2), and saponins (e.g., platycodin D).

Common Antiviral Compounds in Medicinal Herbs Used for SARS-CoV-1, SARS-CoV-2, et al. Viral Respiratory Illnesses	
• Berberine	• Huang Qin (Scutellaria Baicalensis), Coptidis Rhizoma (Huang Lian), Rheum Palmatum (Da Huang)
• Flavonoids: Baicalin, Baicalein, Scutellarin. Scutellarein, Wogonin, Chrysin, Oroxylin A	• Huang Qin (Scutellaria Baicalensis)
• Flavonoids: Kaempferol • Quercetin • Apigenin • Luteolin	• Mian Ma Guan Zhong (Dryopteris Crassirhizoma) • Xiang Chun Ye (Toona Sinensis Roem) • Jin Yin Hua (Flos Lonicerae Japonicae) • Zi Hua Di Ding (Herba Violae)
• Anthraquinones - Emodin	• Da Huang (Rheum Palmatum)
• Polysaccharides	• Yu Xing Cao (Houttuynia Cordata)
• Saikosaponin B2	• Chai Hu (Radix Bupleuri), Xuan Shen (Scrophularia Scorodonia)
• Saponins - Platycodin D	• Jie Geng (Radix Platycodi)
• Terpenoids – Glycyrrhizin • Artemisinin	• Gan Cao (Radix Glycyrrhizae) • Qing Hao (Artemisia Annua)
• Resveratrol	• Hu Zhang (Rhizoma Polygoni Cuspidati)
• Phenylpropanoids: • Chlorogenic acid	• Huo Xiang (Herba Pogostemonis) • Jin Yin Hua (Flos Lonicerae Japonicae),

	• Zi Wan (Radix et Rhizoma Asteris)
• Phenolic acids • Ferulic acid	• Hong Jing Tian (Radix et Rhizoma Rhodiola Crenulata) • She Gan (Rhizoma Belamcandae)

These compounds (combined in herbal formulas) have proven empirically effective for a broad spectrum of viruses throughout centuries of use, including during other epidemics such as SARS-CoV-1 in 2002, which inspires hope that they may be similarly useful for the current SARS-CoV-2 pandemic. Keep these compounds in mind as you read through this text and start identifying the herbs that contain them.

While there is still no scientific proof that these compounds are clinically useful for Covid-19 patients via randomized, double-blind, placebo-controlled trials, we will investigate the possibility that the same compounds that have inhibited homologous coronaviruses like SARS-CoV-1, may also be useful for SARS-CoV-2.

IMPORTANT POLYPHENOLS AND PHYTOCHEMICALS

This book will establish the role of polyphenols and other phytochemicals that act as antiviral, immune-modulating, and anti-inflammatory agents. Phytochemicals are considered to be essential for optimal health and disease prevention (Ballantyne, 2017). The term polyphenols describe a larger category of approximately 8000 phytochemicals, including flavonoids, phenolic acids, and lignans in fruits, vegetables, and medicinal herbs that act as micronutrients (Azam et al., 2019). Polyphenols have a molecular structure with multiple OH groups around their periphery, which allow them to impact numerous cellular functions, including immune function (Ding et al., 2018). For example, herbs that contain polyphenols may help modulate upstream (TLR activation) and downstream kinase (MAPK) and transcription factors (NFKB) pathways to reduce proinflammatory cytokines (Azam et al., 2019). Importantly, many of the herbs and foods containing these compounds have multiple beneficial functions, including antiviral, immune-modulating, and anti-inflammatory effects, which make them excellent candidates for viral respiratory infections.

FUNCTIONAL FLAVONOIDS

Flavonoids are polyphenolic substances that make up the plant pigments found in fruits, vegetables, and medicinal herbs, which have numerous biological properties, including antimicrobial, anti-inflammatory, and immune-modulating effects (Lago et al., 2014). Flavonoids are categorized into flavonols, flavones, flavanones, isoflavones, flavon-3-ols, catechins, anthocyanidins, and chalcones (ibid, 2014). The potent therapeutic effects of these polyphenolic substances are directly associated with their capacity to donate hydrogen radicals from their phenolic groups (Ding et al., 2018).

Flavonoids are ubiquitous in Chinese herbs and have been extensively investigated for viral respiratory infections (Patel et al., 2018; Eng et al., 2019; Huang et al., 2020; Zakarayan et al., 2017; Ding et al., 2018). A recent virtual screening study showed that flavonoids, including hesperidin, baicalin, kaempferol, and rutin, may also effectively interact with targets of SARS-CoV-2 (Wu et al., 2020). Intriguingly, in a molecular docking study, Khaerunnisa et al. (2020) found that the most potent antiviral flavonoids predicted to inhibit the main protease (M^{pro}) in SARS-CoV-2 are kaempferol, luteolin, and quercetin. Below are charts of herbs used routinely for respiratory infections that contain each of the flavonoids, kaempferol, luteolin, and quercetin. Pay attention to the herbs that contain multiple antiviral flavonoids.

Common Antiviral Flavonoids in Medicinal Herbs Used for SARS-CoV-1, SARS-CoV-2, et al. Viral Respiratory Illnesses	
Herbs That Contain Kaempferol	
<ul><li>Sang Ye (Folium Mori)</li><li>Mian Ma Guan Zhong (Dryopteris Crassirhizoma)</li><li>Ma Huang (Herba Ephedrae)</li><li>Huang Qi (Astragalus Membranaceus)</li><li>Lian Qiao (Fructus Forsythiae)</li><li>Pi Pa Ye (Eriobotryae Folium)</li></ul>	<ul><li>Jin Yin Hua (Flos Lonicerae Japonicae)</li><li>Ju Hua (Flos Chrysanthemi)</li><li>Bo He (Herba Menthae)</li><li>Hong Jing Tian (Radix et Rhizoma Rhodiola Crenulata)</li></ul>
Herbs That Contain Quercetin	
<ul><li>Xiang Chun Ye (Toona Sinensis Roem)</li><li>Ma Huang (Herba Ephedrae)</li><li>Zi Hua Di Ding (Herba Violae)</li><li>Bo He (Herba Menthae)</li><li>Hu Zhang (Rhizoma Polygoni Cuspidati)</li><li>Jin Yin Hua (Flos Lonicerae Japonicae)</li><li>Pi Pa Ye (Eriobotryae Folium)</li></ul>	<ul><li>Lian Qiao (Fructus Forsythiae)</li><li>Yu Xing Cao (Houttuynia Cordata)</li><li>Ju Hua (Flos Chrysanthemi)</li><li>Sang Ye (Folium Mori)</li><li>Zi Wan (Radix et Rhizoma Asteris)</li><li>Hong Jing Tian (Radix et Rhizoma Rhodiola Crenulata)</li><li>Xiang Ru (Herba Moslae)</li></ul>

Herbs That Contain Luteolin	
• Xiang Ru (Herba Moslae) • Ju Hua (Flos Chrysanthemi) • Ma Huang (Herba Ephedrae) • Zi Hua Di Ding (Herba Violae) • Hong Jing Tian (Radix Rhodiola Crenulata)	• Lian Qiao (Fructus Forsythiae) • Jin Yin Hua (Flos Lonicerae Japonicae) • Yu Xing Cao (Houttuynia Cordata)

Terpenoids

Terpenoids are a class of hydrocarbons, including terpenes, diterpenes, triterpenes, and sesquiterpenes that have been identified as antiviral, antibacterial, antifungal, and immunomodulatory agents (Brahkshatriya et al., 2013). Terpenoids refer to plant compounds before they are oxidized, while terpenes refer to the volatile oils that comprise the scent of a plant. Terpenoids in Chinese medicinal herbs have been extensively studied for acute lung injury (ALI) and acute respiratory distress syndrome (ARDS). Acute lung injury (ALI) is characterized by pulmonary edema and diffuse alveolar damage (DAD), which can cause acute progressive respiratory distress and persistent hypoxemia (Ding et al., 2020). Acute respiratory distress syndrome (ARDS) is a severe progression of ALI, as seen in some cases of Covid-19.

The terpenoid asatone, from the dried roots and rhizomes of Xi Xin (Radix et Rhizoma Asari), has been shown to help prevent acute lung injury by reducing NFKB and MAPK signaling pathways in vitro (Chang et al., 2018). Xi Xin is one of the herbs in *Qing Fei Pai Du Tang*, i.e., the most recommended formula for pneumonia in Covid-19 patients in China (see below).

Qing Hao (Artemisia Annua) also contains a sesquiterpene lactone, artemisinin, known for its anti-inflammatory and antimalarial effects (Ivanescu et al., 2015). Qing Hao is often included in remedies for influenza and other viral infections

(Efferth, 2018). Interestingly, sources of sesquiterpene lactones in our diet include lettuce, chicory, and star anise (Chadwick et al., 2013).

Andrographolide is a diterpenoid derivative from Andrographis Paniculata (Chuan Xin Lian), which is predicted to inhibit 3CL^{pro} and helicase proteins in SARS-CoV-2 (Wu et al., 2020). Gan Cao (Radix Glycyrrhizae) contains the triterpenoid saponin, glycyrrhizin, which demonstrates antiviral properties against SARS-CoV-1 and SARS-CoV-2 (Cinatl et al., 2003; Song et al., 2014; Chen & Du, 2020). Glycyrrhizin also inhibits lipopolysaccharide (LPS) induced cytokine expression of IL-6 in murine macrophages (Liu et al., 2014).

The above terpenoids exhibit multiple actions, including viral inhibition along with modulation of NFKB and cytokines. These are just a few examples of the potent terpenoids in traditional Chinese herbs that point toward their usefulness for viral respiratory illnesses.

Saikosaponins

Saikosaponins are naturally occurring triterpene glycosides in medicinal herbs that have known antiviral effects. For example, in 2006, Cheng et al. showed that saikosaponin B2 (from herbs such as Bupleurum [Chai Hu] and Scrophularia Scorodonia [Xuan Shen]) has antiviral effects, such as inhibition of viral attachment and penetration of both human coronavirus HCoV-22E9 (a species of CoV known to cause mild to moderate respiratory infections), and HCoV-OC43, which is one of the viruses responsible for the common cold.

Saponins

Saponins are naturally occurring compounds that have many studied health benefits. Chemically speaking, saponins contain a carbohydrate moiety attached to a triterpenoid or steroid (Shi et al., 2004). Saponins are also important anti-inflammatory agents in plants that can be considered for acute lung injury (ALI) and acute respiratory distress syndrome (ARDS).

Saponins inhibit the release of pro-inflammatory factors and related proteins (De Costa et al., 2011). For example, ginsenosides Rg1 derived from Panax Ginseng has been shown to improve lipopolysaccharide (LPS) induced acute lung injury by inhibiting inflammatory responses and modulating infiltration of M2 macrophages (Bao et al., 2015). Ginsenoside Rg1 also regulates innate immune responses in macrophages through differentially modulating the NFKB and PI3K/Akt/mTOR signaling pathways important for regulating the cell cycle (Wang et al., 2014).

The saponin, platycodin D, in the dried roots of Platycodon Grandiflorum (Jie Geng), decreases caspase-3 (a protein that is activated upon the initiation of apoptosis) thereby inhibiting lung epithelial cell apoptosis and inflammation in (LPS induced) acute lung injury (Tao et al., 2015).

Polysaccharides

Plant polysaccharides from Houttuynia Cordata (Yu Xing Cao) were shown to reduce pulmonary edema, protein exudation, and the deposition of complement activation products, thereby mitigating acute lung injury in rats (Lu et al., 2018). Astragalus polysaccharides have also been shown to exert immunomodulatory effects via the TLR4-mediated MyD88-dependent signaling pathway in vitro and in vivo (Zhou et al., 2017). This is significant as it is speculated that the TLR4/MyD88 signaling pathway is related to the activation of macrophages and inflammatory factors in ARDS (Zhou et al., 2018).

The Simple Takeaway
The synergistic effects of these plant compounds are especially potent when combined in remedies. With this understanding, let's review herbs that are used routinely in formulas for viral respiratory infections.

HERBS FOR VIRAL RESPIRATORY INFECTIONS

Bioactive plant compounds such as flavonoids, saikosaponins, saponins, and terpenoids are abundant in the most commonly used herb formulas chosen for viral respiratory infections. Many studies reveal that these potent plant compounds have multiple therapeutic functions, including antiviral, immune-modulating, and anti-inflammatory effects (Zakarayan et al., 2017; Ding et al., 2018).

A recent computer modeling study by Zhang et al., (2020) revealed several natural compounds, in Chinese herbs used for viral respiratory infections, that had a high probability of directly inhibiting viral entry and replication of SARS-CoV-2 via the spike protein or proteases, PL^{pro} and 3CL^{pro}. The following chart lists all of the natural compounds and the viral targets that they interfere with.

Antiviral Compounds in Herbs Routinely Used for Respiratory Infections That Target SARS-CoV-2
- Kaempferol (PL^{pro} and 3CL^{pro})
- Quercetin (PL^{pro} and 3CL^{pro})
- Betulinic acid (Replication, 3CL^{pro})
- Coumaroyltyramine (PL^{pro} and 3CL^{pro})
- Cryptotanshinone (PL^{pro} and 3CL^{pro})
- Desmethoxyreserpine (Entry, Replication, 3CL^{pro})
- Dihomo-γ-linolenic acid (3CL^{pro})
- Dihydrotanshinone (Entry, and spike protein)
- Lignan (Replication, 3CL^{pro})
- Moupinamide (PL^{pro})
- N-cis-feruloyltyramine (PL^{pro} and 3CL^{pro})
- Sugiol (Replication, 3CL^{pro})
- Tanshinone IIa (PL^{pro} and 3CL^{pro})

Network pharmacology analysis of the following herbs shows that they contain at least two or more of these compounds related to regulating viral infection, immune-inflammation reactions, and hypoxia response (ibid, 2020).

Herbs Routinely Used for Viral Respiratory Infections That Contain 2 or More Antiviral Compounds	
• Lian Qiao (Forsythiae Fructus) • Gan Cao (Radix Glycyrrhizae) • Sang Ye (Folium Mori) • Sang Bai Pi (Mori Cortex) • Ju Hua (Flos Chrysanthemi) • Jin Yin Hua (Flos Lonicerae Japonicae) • Pi Pa Ye (Eriobotryae Folium) • Zi Wan (Radix et Rhizoma Asteris) • Kuan Dong Hua (Flos Farfarae) • Bai Guo (Ginkgo Biloba Semen) • Xi Xin (Radix et Rhizoma Asari)	• Chai Hu (Radix Bupleuri) • Huang Qin (Scutellaria Baicalensis) • Huang Lian (Coptidis Rhizoma) • Yu Xing Cao (Houttuynia Cordata) • Ting Li Zi (Semen Lepidii) • Qian Hu (Peucedani Radix) • Xuan Fu Hua (Flos Inulae) • Zhi Mu (Rhizoma Anemarrhenae)

These are the precise medicinal herbs that are commonly recommended for various viral respiratory illnesses, including Covid-19 in China. This research points to the potential benefits of herbal medicine for viral respiratory infections in general and the possibility that they may be useful for SARS-CoV-2. While we still do not have human studies to affirm the most effective herbal formulas for Covid-19 patients, we will review the bioactive compounds in herbs and formulas used for other viral respiratory infections (including SARS-CoV-1) and some of the current formulas now being recommended for SARS-CoV-2.

SARS-COV-2 GENOMICS, TRANSMISSION, AND RISK FACTORS

Severe acute respiratory syndrome coronavirus 2 (SARS-CoV-2) is an enveloped, positive-sense, single-stranded RNA virus that causes Covid-19 (Pal et al., 2020). SARS-CoV-2 belongs to the genus Betacoronavirus, which also includes SARS-CoV-1 and MERS-CoV. SARS-CoV-2 is genetically related to SARS-CoV-1 of the 2002 outbreak (Chen et al., 2020). Sequence analysis of 11 samples found that SARS-CoV-1 and SARS-CoV-2 are 94.6% similar in amino acid sequences across the genome (Zhou et al., 2020).

The human-to-human spread of SARS-CoV-2 has been confirmed via respiratory droplets and aerosols that release while coughing or sneezing (World Health Organization Website, March 29, 2020). There are reports of transmission in the absence of symptoms, and infected people are likely most contagious while coughing and sneezing, which projects respiratory droplets and aerosols (ibid, March 29, 2020). According to the CDC website, the suspected incubation period can be 2-14 days with a median of 4-5 days (June 2, 2020). Symptoms of Covid-19 can include fever, chills, cough, shortness of breath or dyspnea, sore throat, fatigue, myalgia, headache, loss of taste or smell, runny nose or congestion, nausea, vomiting, and diarrhea (ibid, 2020).

According to the latest CDC report on June 25, 2020, an updated list of those at increased risk for severe illness from Covid-19 included people of any age with the following underlying medical conditions: obesity (body mass index [BMI] of 30 or higher), COPD, type II diabetes, serious heart conditions (such as heart failure, coronary artery disease, or cardiomyopathies), chronic kidney disease, Sickle cell disease, and immunocompromised state (weakened immune system) from solid organ transplants (CDC, 2020).

Currently, there is no vaccine, and there are no FDA approved medicines for the treatment of Covid-19 except for emergency use of medications such as Remdesivir for hospitalized patients with severe symptoms (Food and Drug Administration, 2020; National Institute of Health, 2020). With this basic understanding, let's review the research regarding the repurposing of potent antiviral herb compounds for SARS-CoV-2.

VIRAL TARGETS FOR SARS-COV-2 INHIBITION

During and after the SARS-CoV-1 epidemic, scientists identified multiple compounds in traditional Chinese herbs that demonstrated anti-SARS-CoV-1 activity. In 2003, Cinatl et al. showed that the triterpenoid saponin, glycyrrhizin, derived from Gan Cao (Glycyrrhiza Glabra), potently inhibited viral replication in SARS-CoV-1, making it a viable resource for drug development. Currently, the search is on for other potent antiviral compounds that are effective against SARS-CoV-2. In the same way that Western doctors search for the best antiviral pharmaceuticals, researchers are also looking at plant compounds in medicinal herbs that show antiviral activity in terms of blocking entry and interrupting replication.

For herbs to be considered effective antivirals against SARS-CoV-2, they must interfere with the viral attachment, entry, and replication process. A novel antiviral herbal formula would ideally act on all levels to inhibit the damaging effects of SARS-CoV-2. As you read through each section, pay attention to the compounds that have antiviral effects on multiple pathways.

Some of the pathways that we will explore include:
1. ACE2 blockade
2. $3CL^{pro}$ (M^{pro}) inhibition
3. PL^{pro} inhibition
4. Spike protein binding
5. Helicase inhibition
6. RNA- dependent RNA polymerase (RdRp) inhibition

7. Viroporin 3a ion channel inhibition
8. TMPRSS2 inhibition

To learn more about herb compounds that may inhibit viral attachment, entry, and replication, let's continue with a review of each target.

ACE2 BLOCKADE

Once Hoffmann et al. (2020) confirmed that the angiotensin-converting enzyme 2 (ACE2) is the cellular receptor for SARS-CoV-2, as it is for SARS-CoV-1, researchers started considering that the same active compounds which blocked ACE2 in SARS-CoV-1, might also prevent SARS-CoV-2 from attaching to ACE2.

In 2007, researchers Ho et al. demonstrated that Emodin from genus Rheum Palmatum (Da Huang), and Polygonum Multiflorum (He Shou Wu) markedly inhibited the interaction of SARS-CoV-1 Spike (S) protein and ACE2. Emodin is a natural anthraquinone (diterpenoid) derivative found in many medicinal herbs, such as Rheum Palmatum (Da Huang), Polygonum Cuspidatum (Hu Zhang), and Polygonum Multiflorum (He Shou Wu). Emodin is also a known virucidal agent (Alves et al., 2004). Because emodin inhibited the interaction of the SARS-CoV-1 S-protein and ACE2, it is not surprising to see herbs that contain emodin, namely Da Huang (Rheum Palmatum), in an antiviral formula currently being used for Covid-19 in China (see *Lian Hua Qing Wen Capsule* below).

Niu et al. (2020) performed a molecular docking analysis on Chinese herbal formulas commonly used during SARS-CoV-1 and the current formulas recommended in the Covid-19 clinical guidelines. The results found 46 compounds that were predicted to act on the S-protein binding site of ACE2 (Chan et al., 2020). Niu et al. (2020) recommended seven herbs where these compounds are mainly found, including Jin Yin Hua (Flos Lonicerae

Japonicae), Sang Ye (Folium Mori), Cang Zhu (Atractylodes Lancea), Zhe Bei Mu (Bulbus Fritillariae Thunbergii), Sheng Jiang (Rhizoma Zingiberis Recens), Lian Qiao (Fructus Forsythiae), and Cao Guo (Fructus Amomi Tsaoko) (ibid, 2020).

Chen and Du (2020) have also recently found, through molecular docking techniques, that antiviral constituents including scutellarin from Erigeron Breviscapus (Deng Zhan Hua), baicalin from Scutellaria Baicalensis (Huang Qin), hesperetin from Pericarpium Citri Reticulatae (Chen Pi), glycyrrhizin (Gan Cao), and nicotianamine in soybean may all bind to ACE2 to block entry of SARS-CoV-2 and are predicted to inhibit infection.

Also, the patchouli alcohol in Guang Huo Xiang (Herba Pogostemonis) was found to act on the ACE2 receptor to prevent viral entry (Wu et al., 2020). This research suggests that the herbs containing these compounds may have the potential to inhibit SARS-CoV-2 infection directly. Please note that all of the following herbs are part of formulas that are routinely used for viral respiratory illnesses, including Covid-19 in China (see below).

| Compounds That Might Act on the ACE2 Receptor in SARS-CoV-2 |||
Medicinal Herbs	Bioactive Compounds	Formulas for Covid-19
	Baicalin and Scutellarin (Huang Qin)	*Qing Fei Pai Du Tang* *Chai Ge Jie Ji Tang* *Shuang Huang Lian* Modified *Yu Ping Feng San*

	Hesperetin in Pericarpium Citri Reticulatae (Chen Pi)	*Qing Fei Pai Du Tang* *Huo Xiang Zheng Qi Wan*
	Nicotianamine from soybean (Dan Dou Chi)	*Yin Qiao San*
	Emodin from genus Rheum Palmatum (Da Huang)	*Lian Hua Qing Wen Capsule*
	Glycyrrhizin from Radix Glycyrrhizae (Gan Cao)	*Lian Hua Qing Wen Capsule* *Qing Fei Pai Du Tang* *Yin Qiao San*

	Flos Lonicerae Japonicae (Jin Yin Hua) Flavonoids: Luteolin, kaempferol, quercetin, apigenin, rutin, caffeic acid, chlorogenic acid, lonicerin (Xu et al., 2019).	*Lian Hua Qing Wen Capsule* *Yin Qiao San* Modified *Ge Gen Tang* Modified *Yu Ping Feng San*
	Folium Mori (Sang Ye) Flavonoids: Rutin, isoquercitrin, astragalin, kaempferol, quercetin, chlorogenic acid (Zhang et al., 2017). Quercetin, kaempferol, rutin, morin (Chen et al., 2018). Rutin, isoquercitrin, astragalin, gallic acid (Kim et al., 2014).	*Sang Ju Yin* Modified *Yu Ping Feng San*
	Fructus Forsythiae (Lian Qiao) Flavonoids: Luteolin, quercetin, kaempferol, rutin, baicalin, wogonin. Lignans (forsythin)	*Lian Hua Qing Wen Capsule* *Yin Qiao San* Modified *Yu Ping Feng San*

	triterpenoids (betulinic acid, oleanolic acid, ursolic acid) (Dong et al., 2017).	
	Patchouli alcohol in Herba Pogostemonis (Guang Huo Xiang)	*Huo Xiang Zheng Qi Wan* *Qing Fei Pai Du Tang* Modified *Yu Ping Feng San*
	Cang Zhu (Atractylodes Lancea) Sesquiterpenes, sesquiterpenoids, polyethylene alkynes, phytosterols, elemol, β-selinene and atractylone (Zhang et al., 2012).	Modified *Yu Ping Feng San*
	Zhe Bei Mu (Bulbus Fritillariae Thunbergii) Steroidal alkaloids, saponins, terpenoids, glycosides (Hao et al., 2009). Antitussive Antiasthmatic Expectorant (Hao et al., 2013).	*Sha Shen Mai Dong Tang*

	Cao Guo (Fructus Amomi Tsaoko) Flavonoids: Quercetin, Isoquercetin. Volatile oils: Bornyl acetate, camphor, borneol, camphene, alpha-pinene, beta-pinene and alpha copaene (Xiao et al., 2020).	Modified *Yu Ping Feng San*
	Sheng Jiang (Rhizoma Zingiberis Recens) Gingerol, allicin, and shogaol (Eng et al., 2019). Allicin in ginger (Zingiber officinale) inhibits influenza A (H1N1) neuraminidase (Sahoo et al., 2016).	*Qing Fei Pai Du Tang* *Ge Gen Tang* *Chai Ge Jie Ji Tang* *Xiao Chai Hu Tang* *She Gan Ma Huang Tang*

The fact that many of these compounds target ACE2 holds the promise that they may also be useful for inhibiting SARS-CoV-2 infection. Also, techniques like molecular docking analysis and virtual screening research allow us to consider our herbal formulations in a new way.

Other Targets

The coronavirus encodes many proteins, including the most well studied main protease, M^{Pro}, (also known as 3C-like protease (3CL^{Pro}), papain-like protease (PL^{Pro}), and the Spike (S)-protein. Herb compounds that interrupt or inhibit these enzymes and, therefore, viral attachment and replication will now be explored.

3CL^{PRO}/M^{PRO} INHIBITION

SARS-CoV-2 like SARS-CoV-1 is an enveloped positive-sense single-stranded RNA virus that encodes two proteases for proteolytic processing: a papain-like protease (PL^{Pro}) and the main protease M^{Pro}, i.e., the chymotrypsin-like cysteine protease (3C-like protease; 3CL^{Pro}) (Pal et al., 2020; Rota et al., 2003). To get clear on the terms, the main protease M^{Pro} is also known as 3CL^{Pro} and will be used interchangeably, depending on the study referenced. 3CL^{Pro} is a key CoV enzyme that plays an important role in mediating viral replication and transcription (Jin et al., 2020). 3CL^{Pro} is individually responsible for releasing critical replicative enzymes such as RdRp and helicase from polyprotein precursors (Thiel et al., 2011).

Because 3- chymotrypsin-like cysteine protease (3CL^{Pro}) is so important for viral replication, it was considered as a drug target for the development of therapeutics agents for SARS-CoV-1 (Grum-Tokars et al., 2008) and is now being considered for SARS-CoV-2 (Wu et al., 2020, Zhang et al., 2020; Khaerunnisa et al., 2020). The following herbal extracts have antiviral effects against SARS-CoV-1, including inhibiting the activity of the main protease in SARS-CoV-1 3CL^{Pro}/M^{Pro}.

1. Rhubarb extracts (Da Haung) (Luo et al., 2009).
2. Flavonoids extracted from litchi seeds (Li Zhi He) (Gong et al., 2008).
3. Phenolic compounds aloe-emodin, hesperetin, and the root extracts of Isatis Indigotica (Ban Lan Gen): sinigrin, β-sitosterol, and indigo, dose-dependently inhibited cleavage activities of the 3CL^{Pro} in cell-free

and cell-based assays (Lin et al., 2015).

4. Quercetin, quercetrin, and cinanserin from the water extract of Houttuynia Cordata (Yu Xing Cao) (Lau et al., 2008). Houttuynia Cordata (Yu Xing Cao) extracts inhibit 3CL^{pro} in SARS-CoV-1 (Fung, 2011).

5. Flavonoids, including apigenin, luteolin, quercetin, amentoflavone, daidzein, puerarin, epigallocatechin, epigallocatechin gallate, gallocatechin gallate, and kaempferol (Nguyen et al., 2012; Schwarz et al., 2014; Jo et al., 2020).

6. The flavonol, herbacetin, and two flavones, rhoifolin and pectolinarin have also been shown to inhibit the protease activity of SARS-CoV-1 3CL^{pro} (Jo et al., 2020).

All of these compounds inhibited the proteolytic activity of 3CL^{pro} in SARS-CoV-1, suggesting that they all may be promising candidates for 3CL^{pro} inhibition in SARS-CoV-2. Wu et al., (2004) also found that the saponin, ginsenoside-Rb1 (from Panax Ginseng), extracts of eucalyptus, and Flos Lonicerae Japonicae (Jin Yin Hua) all exhibited antiviral activity against SARS-CoV-1 replication.

Recent virtual screening research shows that patchouli alcohol contained in Guang Huo Xiang (Herba Pogostemonis) also inhibits 3CL^{pro} and, therefore, viral replication of SARS-CoV-2 (Wu et al., 2020). Wu et al., (2020), also discovered that andrographolide (a diterpenoid) derivatives from Andrographis Paniculata (Chuan Xin Lian), chrysin-7-O-β-glucuronide from Scutellaria Baicalensis (Huang Qin), 2β-hydroxy-3,4-seco-friedelolactone-27-oic acid, isodecortinol and cerevisterol from Viola Diffusa (Zi Hua Di Ding), hesperidin and neohesperidin from Citrus Aurantium (Zhi Shi), and xanthones (kouitchenside I and deacetylcentapicrin) from the plants of Swertia genus (Gentianaceae) all demonstrate potential as 3CL^{pro} inhibitors that could be used for SARS-CoV-2. Mian Ma Guan Zhong (Dryopteris Crassirhizoma) contains kaempferol, which inhibits both $3CL^{pro}$ and PL^{pro} and shows the potential to inhibit SARS-CoV-2 (Zhang et al., 2020).

Also, there is one preprint molecular docking study that ranked both drugs and natural compounds that may be useful for inhibiting the main protease M^{pro} in SARS-CoV-2 (Khaerunnisa et al., 2020). Khaerunnisa et al. (2020) showed that herbal compounds such as kaempferol, quercetin, luteolin-7-glucoside, demethoxycurcumin, naringenin, apigenin-7-glucoside, oleuropein, curcumin, catechin, and epicatechin-gallate were all predicted to act as potential inhibitors of SARS-CoV-2 $3CL^{pro}/M^{pro}$. Interestingly, kaempferol, quercetin, and luteolin-7-glucoside all formed chemical bonds similar to Nelfinavir while luteolin-7-glucoside and kaempferol compounds were predicted to play binding roles at the active site of SARS-CoV-2 $3CL^{pro}/M^{pro}$ (ibid, 2020).

Compounds That Might Target $3CL^{pro}/M^{pro}$ in SARS-CoV-2		
Medicinal Herbs	Bioactive Compounds and Actions	Covid-19 Formulas
	Root extracts from Isatis Indigotica (Ban Lan Gen) Sinigrin, β-sitosterol, and Indigo inhibit $3CL^{pro}$ in SARS-CoV-1 (Lin et al., 2015).	*Lian Hua Qing Wen Capsule* Modified *Yu Ping Feng San*
	Rhubarb extracts from Rheum Palmatum (Da Huang) inhibit $3CL^{pro}$ in SARS-CoV-1 (Luo et al., 2009).	*Lian Hua Qing Wen Capsule*

	Puerarin and Daidzein (Ge Gen) Flavonoids puerarin and daidzein inhibit 3CL^{pro} in SARS-CoV-1 (Nguyen, et al., 2012; Schwarz et al., 2014).	*Ge Gen Tang* *Chai Ge Jie Ji Tang*
	Houttuynia Cordata (Yu Xing Cao) extracts inhibit 3CL^{pro} in SARS-CoV-1 (Fung, 2011). Quercetin, quercetrin, and cinanserin from the water extract of Houttuynia Cordata (Yu Xing Cao) inhibit 3CL^{pro} in SARS-CoV-1 (Lau et al., 2008).	*Qing Fei Pai Du Tang* *Lian Hua Qing Wen Capsule*
	Flavonoids extracted from litchi seeds (Li Zhi He) inhibit 3CL^{pro} in SARS-CoV-1 (Gong et al., 2008).	Extra herb
	Patchouli alcohol contained in Guang Huo Xiang (Herba Pogostemonis) inhibits 3CL^{pro} and, therefore, viral replication of SARS-CoV-2 (Wu et al., 2020).	*Huo Xiang Zheng Qi Wan* *Qing Fei Pai Du Tang*

	Mian Ma Guan Zhong (Dryopteris Crassirhizoma) contains kaempferol, which inhibits both PL^{pro} and 3CL^{pro}, and has the potential to inhibit SARS-CoV-2 (Zhang et al., 2020).	*Lian Hua Qing Wen Capsule* Modified *Yu Ping Feng San*
	Fructus Aurantii Immaturus (Zhi Shi) Hesperidin, neohesperidin, hesperetin, rutin, rhoifolin, naringenin (Bai et al., 2018). Hesperidin and neohesperidin demonstrate potential as M^{pro} inhibitors (Khaerunnisa et al., 2020).	*Qing Fe Pai Du Tang*
	Radix Curcumae (Yu Jin) Demethoxycurcumin and curcumin demonstrate potential as M^{pro} inhibitors (Khaerunnisa et al., 2020).	Extra Herb
	Green tea (Lu Cha) Catechin and Epigallocatechin Gallate (EGCG) demonstrate potential as M^{pro} inhibitors (Khaerunnisa et al., 2020).	Extra herb

	Toona Sinensis Roem (Xiang Chun Ye) contains quercetin, gallic acid, kaempferol, rutin, catechin, epicatechin, β-sitosterol, toosendanin, and phytol (Chia et al., 2007). Quercetin demonstrates potential for M^{pro} inhibition in SARS-CoV-2 (Khaerunnisa et al., 2020). TSL-1 extracted from Toona Sinensis Roem (Xiang Chun Ye) inhibits replication of SARS-CoV-1 (Chen et al., 2008).	Extra Herb
	Flos Lonicerae Japonicae (Jin Yin Hua) Luteolin and apigenin demonstrate potential as M^{pro} inhibitors (Khaerunnisa et al., 2020).	*Lian Hua Qing Wen Capsule* *Yin Qiao San* Modified *Ge Gen Tang* Modified *Yu Ping Feng San*

	Scutellaria Baicalensis (Huang Qin) Chrysin shows potential for 3CL^{pro} inhibition (Wu et al., 2020).	*Qing Fei Pai Du Tang* *Chai Ge Jie Ji Tang* *Shuang Huang Lian* Modified *Yu Ping Feng San*
	Swertia genus (Gentianaceae) Radix Gentianae Macrophyllae (Qin Jiao) Xanthones: kouitchenside I and deacetylcentapicrin demonstrate potential as 3CL^{pro} inhibitors (Wu et al., 2020). Kouitchenside I and deacetylcentapicrin also demonstrate potential as helicase inhibitors (Wu et al., 2020).	Extra Herb

| | Andrographis Paniculata (Chuan Xin Lian)

Andrographolide, apigenin, luteolin (Rafi et al., 2020).

Andrographolide is predicted to inhibit 3CL^{pro} and helicase proteins in SARS-CoV-2 (Wu et al., 2020). | *Chuan Xin Lian Wan* |
|---|---|---|
| | Viola Diffusa (Zi Hua Di Ding)

Luteolin, quercetin, anthocyanin.

2β-hydroxy-3,4-seco-friedelolactone-27-oic acid, isodecortinol, and cerevisterol demonstrate potential as 3CL^{pro} inhibitors (Wu et al., 2020). | Extra Herb |

PL^PRO INHIBITION

In their virtual screening study, Wu et al. (2020) found naturally derived compounds with the highest binding affinity to papain-like protease (PL^pro) in SARS-CoV-2 including:

- The saponin, platycodin D, from Platycodon Radix (Jie Geng)
- Baicalin from Scutellaria Baicalensis (Huang Qin)
- Sugetriol-3, 9-diacetate from Cyperus Rotundus (Xiang Fu)
- Phaitanthrin D and 2,2-di (3-indolyl)-3-indolone from Isatis Indigotica (Ban Lan Gen)
- Catechin compounds and epigallocatechin gallate from green tea (Lu Cha)

All of these compounds demonstrated a high binding affinity to PL^pro, suggesting the potential utility of these compounds to inhibit PL^pro in SARS-CoV-2. Computer modeling by Zhang et al. (2020) showed that kaempferol, which is contained in Mian Ma Guan Zhong, inhibits both 3CL^pro and PL^pro, and has the potential to inhibit SARS-CoV-2.

Compounds That Might Target PL^pro in SARS-CoV-2		
Medicinal Herbs	Bioactive Compounds and Actions	Formulas for Covid-19
	Phaitanthrin D and 2,2-di (3-indolyl)-3-indolone from Isatis Indigotica (Ban Lan Gen) has a high binding affinity to PL^pro in SARS-CoV-2 (Wu et al., 2020).	*Qing Fei Pai Du Tang* *Lian Hua Qing Wen Capsule*

	Sugetriol-3,9-diacetate in Cyperus Rotundus (Xiang Fu) has a high binding affinity to PL^{pro} in SARS-CoV-2 (Wu et al., 2020).	Extra herb
	Baicalin in Scutellaria Baicalensis (Huang Qin) has a high binding affinity to PL^{pro} in SARS-CoV-2 (Wu et al., 2020).	*Qing Fei Pai Du Tang* *Lian Hua Qing Wen Capsule* *Chai Ge Jie Ji Tang*
	Platycodin D in Platycodon Radix (Jie Geng) has a high binding affinity to PL^{pro} in SARS-CoV-2 (Wu et al., 2020).	*Qing Fei Pai Du Tang* *Yin Qiao San*
	Catechin and epigallocatechin gallate from green tea (Lu Cha) has a high binding affinity to PL^{pro} in SARS-CoV-2 (Wu et al., 2020).	Extra herb

	Kaempferol in Mian Ma Guan Zhong (Dryopteris Crassirhizoma) inhibits both PL^{pro} and 3CL^{pro}, and has the potential to inhibit SARS-CoV-2 (Zhang et al., 2020).	*Lian Qua Qing Wen Capsule* *Modified Yu Ping Feng San*

SPIKE PROTEIN BINDING

Of the four structural proteins in coronaviruses, including spike (S), envelope (E), membrane (M), and nucleocapsid (N) proteins, the S-protein plays the most important role in viral attachment, fusion, and entry (Wang et al., 2016). After the spike of SARS-CoV-1 is cleaved into S1 and S2 by the host cell protease (TMPRSS2), the primary function of S1 is to bind with host cell surface receptors while S2 is responsible for recognition and fusion of the virus to the host membrane (Xia et al., 2014). The structural integrity and cleavage activation of the spike protein play a key role in coronavirus invasion and virulence (ibid, 2014).

Given the homology of SARS-CoV-1 and SARS-CoV-2, therapeutic strategies to block the novel coronavirus from entering host cells by targeting spike proteins or specific receptors on the host surface is considered to be valuable for the development of antiviral drugs (Wu et al., 2020).

Interestingly, promising compounds such as Tetra-O-galloyl-β-D-glucose (TGG) from Galla Chinensis (Wu Bei Zi) and luteolin extracted from many Chinese herbs have been shown to bind with the surface spike (S2) protein of SARS-CoV-1 to block entry into the host cell (Yi et al., 2004). This research suggests that the herbs containing these compounds may add to the list of potential candidates to explore for SARS-CoV-2.

Luteolin is a flavone found in many medicinal herbs including, Rhodiola species (Hong Jing Tian) (Zuo et al., 2007), Flos Lonicerae Japonicae (Jin Yin Hua) (Avendano et al., 2015), Veronica Linariifolia (Scrophulariaceae family) (Ma et al., 1991), Ju Hua (Flos Chrysanthemi) (Du et al., 2015). Luteolin is also contained in Zi Hua Di Ding (Viola Yedoensis Makino) (Peng et al., 2017), Ma Huang (Herba Ephedrae) (Huang et al., 2020), and Xiang Ru (Herba Moslae) (Hu et al., 2010), among others.

HELICASE INHIBITION

The helicase protein is also considered a target for anti-HCoV (human coronavirus) agents. In 2012, Yu et al. reported that scutellarein and myricetin potently inhibited the nsP13 (SARS-CoV-1 helicase protein) in vitro by affecting ATPase activity. A recent virtual screening study of anti-SARS-CoV-2 compounds revealed that hesperidin, rutin, quercetagetin, xanthones from Swertia genus (Gentianaceae), phyllaemblicin B, and phyllaemblinol from Indian Gooseberry (Phyllanthus Emblica), aka Amla, all have a high binding affinity to the helicase protein (Wu et al., 2020). This research suggests that the following herbs containing these compounds may also contribute to the list of potential candidates to explore for SARS-CoV-2. Please note the formulas for Covid-19 that contain these compounds in the chart below.

Compounds That Might Target the Helicase Protein in SARS-CoV-2		
Medicinal Herbs	Bioactive Compounds and Actions	Covid-19 Formula
	Scutellaria Baicalensis (Huang Qin) Scutellarein inhibits the SARS-CoV-1 helicase protein in vitro (Yu et al., 2012).	*Qing Fei Pai Du Tang* *Chai Ge Jie Ji Tang* *Shuang Huang Lian*
	Swertia genus (Gentianaceae) Radix Gentianae Macrophyllae (Qin Jiao) Xanthones: Kouitchenside I and deacetylcentapicrin demonstrate potential as helicase inhibitors (Wu et al., 2020). Kouitchenside I and deacetylcentapicrin also demonstrate potential as 3CL^{pro} inhibitors (Wu et al., 2020).	Extra Herb

	Andrographis Paniculata (Chuan Xin Lian) Andrographolide, apigeninl, luteolin (Rafi et al., 2020). Andrographolide is predicted to inhibit $3CL^{pro}$ and helicase proteins in SARS-CoV-2 (Wu et al., 2020).	*Chuan XIn Lian Wan*
	Phyllanthus Emblica (Yu Gan Zi) aka Indian Gooseberry (Amla) Phyllaemblicin B and Phyllaemblinol have high binding affinity to the helicase protein in SARS-CoV-2 (Wu et al., 2020).	Extra Herb
	Zhi Shi (Fructus Aurantii Immaturus) Hesperidin, neohesperidin, hesperetin, rutin, rhoifolin, naringenin (Bai et al., 2018). Hesperidin has high binding affinity to the helicase protein in SARS-CoV-2 (Wu et al., 2020).	*Qing Fei Pai Du Tang*

RNA-DEPENDENT RNA POLYMERASE (RDRP) INHIBITION

RNA-dependent RNA polymerase (RdRp) is an enzyme responsible for RNA synthesis, representing another potential target in SARS-CoV-2 as it was for SARS-CoV-1. Interestingly, this is the target of the (newly approved for Covid-19) antiviral drug Remdesivir. There have been a couple of studies done on herbs that inhibited RdRp in SARS-CoV-1. In 2011, Fung et al. published the results of a clinical trial conducted on 80 healthy subjects using *Kwan Du Bu Fei Tang* (a combination of *Sang Ju Yin* and *Yu Ping Feng San* plus Radix Scutellariae [Huang Qin] and Folium Isatidis [Da Qing Ye]) along with Houttuynia Cordata (Yu Xing Cao), Sinomenium Acutum (Qing Feng Teng), Coriolus Versicolor (Yun Zhi), and Ganoderma Lucidum (Rei Shi). After the subjects took the herbal combination for seven days, the results showed an increase in T-lymphocytes, CD8+ suppressor plus cytotoxic T-lymphocytes, CD4+ helper T-lymphocytes, and CD56+ NK cells in those taking the herbal combination. However, elevations of immune markers were generally not observed at day 21 compared to day 7 or 0 [all $P>0.05$] (ibid, 2011).

Antiviral assays also showed that extracts of the above herbs inhibited SARS-CoV-1 RdRp in a dose-dependent manner (Fung et al., 2011). The most potent inhibitory effects in descending order came from Ganoderma Lucidum (Rei Shi), Coriolus Versicolor (Yun Zhi), Houttuynia Cordata (Yu Xing Cao), and *Kwan Du Bu Fei Tang* (ibid, 2011). In 2008, Lau et al. also showed that Houttuynia Cordata (Yu Xing Cao) inhibited RNA-dependent RNA polymerase activity in SARS-CoV-1. This research suggests that all of these herbs may help to inhibit the RNA-dependent RNA polymerase in SARS-CoV-2. It also indicates that an increase in immune markers is consistent with the use of this herbal formula and that these markers return to normal within a few weeks upon cessation of use.

VIROPORIN 3A ION CHANNEL INHIBITION

The SARS-CoV-1 virus encodes for ion-permeable channels that become incorporated into the membrane of infected cells (Wang et al., 2011). Activation of these channels is involved in the process of virus production and release (Lu et al., 2006). Interestingly, emodin (and kaempferol derivatives including juglanin) inhibits the 3a (viral) ion channel of SARS-CoV-1 and could potentially prevent viral release from infected cells (Schwarz et al., 2011; Schwarz et al., 2014). Since Chen et al. (2015) found that the SARS-Coronavirus Viroporin 3a ion channel activates the NLRP3 inflammasome, it makes sense to consider this target in SARS-CoV-2. Notably, emodin from Da Huang (Rheum Palmatum) is in the potent antiviral formula *Lian Hua Qing Wen Capsule* (see below).

TMPRSS2 INHIBITION

Since the type-II transmembrane serine protease (TMPRSS2) enzyme was known to cut the spike to trigger the infection of SARS-CoV-1 and MERS-CoV, it is also considered a possible target for antiviral drug discovery for SARS-CoV-2. In their virtual screening study, Wu et al. (2020) found antiviral compounds such as phyllaemblicin G7 contained in Indian Gooseberry (Amla), neoandrographolide from Andrographis Paniculata (Chuan Xin Lian), and kouitchenside I, a xanthone from the genus Swertia (Gentianaceae), all demonstrated potential as TMPRSS2 inhibitors.

THE SYNERGISTIC EFFECT

Herbs from the Chinese pharmacy contain compounds that have multiple effects, including modulating NFKB and cytokines, decreasing inflammation, improving DNA methylation, and histone modification (Guo et al., 2016). There are a few herbs that contain multiple compounds that potentiate their synergistic effects in formulas. Gan Cao (Radix Glycyrrhizae) contains the antiviral triterpenoid saponin, glycyrrhizin, which is predicted to bind with the ACE2 receptor to block SARS-CoV-2 entry (Chen & Du, 2020). At the same time, isoliquiritigenin, a flavonoid from Gan Cao, has been shown to inhibit NFKB activation, which suppresses inflammation in acute respiratory distress syndrome (ARDS) (Lago et al., 2014). The therapeutic value of Gan Cao (Radix Glycyrrhizae) makes it a stellar candidate for viral respiratory infections in general, and SARS-CoV-2 in particular.

Another example is Huang Qin (Scutellaria Baicalensis), which contains many active ingredients. Huang Qin contains the flavonoids baicalin, chrysin, wogonin, and oroxylin A, which have demonstrated therapeutic efficacy against acute lung injury (ALI) caused by the influenza A (H1N1) virus (Zhi et al., 2019). Scutellarin is another active antiviral flavonoid in Huang Qin that suppresses NLP3 inflammasome activation in macrophages, decreases NFKB, IL-6, TNF-α, and IL-1β (Liu et al., 2018; Wang et al., 2016; Tan et al., 2016). Scutellarin also protects against lipopolysaccharide-induced acute lung injury via inhibition of NFKB activation (Tan et al., 2009).

Through molecular docking techniques, Chen and Du (2020) show that the flavonoid baicalin, from Scutellaria Baicalensis (Huang Qin), binds with ACE2 to block entry of SARS-CoV-2 and is predicted to inhibit infection. Also, another flavonoid in Huang Qin, scutellarein, was found to inhibit the Helicase protein in SARS-CoV-1 (Yu et al., 2012).

In 2008, Chen et al. showed that TSL-1 extracted from Toona Sinensis Roem, aka Cedrela Sinensis (Xiang Chun Ye), had potent antiviral effects via inhibiting replication of SARS-CoV-1 in vitro. TSL-1 is a fraction of crude extract from the tender leaf of Toona Sinensis Roem (Chen et al., 2008). Toona Sinensis Roem (Xiang Chun Ye) also contains quercetin, gallic acid, kaempferol, rutin, catechin, epicatechin, β-sitosterol, toosendanin, and phytol (Chia et al., 2007).

The Simple Takeaway
The flavonoids, terpenoids, saponins, saikosaponins, polysaccharides, et al. constituents of medicinal herbs studied for SARS-CoV-1 may also have a synergistic therapeutic effect against SAR-CoV-2. All of these potent antiviral compounds regulate a wide range of signaling pathways, such as NFKB and proinflammatory gene expression, which is necessary to modulate the overexpression of cytokines seen in Covid-19 patients. For Covid-19, it is the combination of these synergistic compounds (in herbal formulas) that may all function together to block or inhibit SARS-CoV-2, decrease NFKB and cytokines, and mitigate inflammation.

With this new understanding of medicinal herbs' synergistic potential, let's review the traditional herbal formulas for viral respiratory infections that contain these plant compounds.

PART II

Review of Herbal Formulas for Viral Respiratory Infections

This book aims to introduce practitioners to the antiviral, immune-modulating, and anti-inflammatory compounds (and their actions) in routinely used formulas for viral respiratory infections. We have established that the herbs used in the Chinese pharmacy provide a rich source of therapeutic agents for viral and respiratory diseases and that medicinal herbs have synergistic effects in formulas. In this section, we will review the compounds in herbal formulas and patent remedies that have historically been used for viral respiratory infections and are currently recommended for Covid-19 patients in China.

While many other herbal formulas can be considered, the formulas described herein reflect the presentations that practitioners are most likely to see in a clinical setting outside of the hospital. This will probably be the patients who seek to support immune function, those who have just been infected and need immediate herbal support, those with mild to moderate lung symptoms that do not require hospitalization, and those recovering from viral respiratory infections who might benefit from supportive herbal therapy.

HERBAL MEDICINE FOR VIRAL EPIDEMICS

Traditional Chinese Medicine has had a 2000-year history of helping to control major epidemics – including the most recent Severe Acute Respiratory Syndrome (SARS)-CoV-1 in 2002. Some of the formulas now being used for the SARS-CoV-2 pandemic date back hundreds of years to the Eastern Han Dynasty (25 CE - 220 CE) texts called the *Shang Han Lun* (On Cold Damage) and the *Jin Gui Yao Lue* (Essential Prescriptions of the Golden Cabinet), compiled by Zhang Zhong Jing during his lifetime (150-219 CE). Other formulas stemmed from the *Wen Bing Tiao Bian* (Systematic Differentiation of Warm Disease) published in 1798 by Wu Tang, aka Wu Ju-Tong (1758-1836).

While a detailed discussion of these ancient texts is beyond this book's scope, we will review the herbal properties of a few featured formulas and patent remedies that have traditionally been used for viral respiratory illnesses and are currently recommended for Covid-19 patients in China. Based on some promising reports of faster recovery times and decreased severity of symptoms such as fatigue, poor appetite, and sore throat, we will also analyze the compounds and effects of the most recommended formula for Covid-19 patients in China, *Qing Fei Pai Du Tang*.

Considering the combination of potent plant compounds that we have been reviewing, herbal formulas as supportive therapy for Covid-19 can potentially yield profound therapeutic benefits. The goal for practitioners is to study the active constituents in these formulas and identify the most effective compounds that may prove to be useful for SARS-CoV-2 and other viral respiratory illnesses. While many possible supportive formulas can be considered for each stage of Covid-19, the most recommended ones that have previously been used for viral respiratory infections over many centuries by Traditional Chinese Medicine (TCM) practitioners will be reviewed. For more information about the vast number of formulas used in each phase of Covid-19 in China, please check the official guidelines currently in the 7th edition (Lau, 2020).

Four Phases of Supportive Care

Since the outbreak of SARS-CoV-2 in December 2019, Traditional Chinese Medicine (TCM) specialists have been recommending four phases of supportive care for Covid-19 in China. It is essential to keep in mind that the following four-phase paradigm may also be considered for other respiratory illnesses, including upper and lower respiratory infections, bronchitis, and pneumonia. The first phase aims to improve host defenses against infection. The second phase addresses the early stage of infection, which may be characterized by fever, sore throat, dry cough, dyspnea, myalgia, digestive distress, and fatigue. The third phase addresses the acute stage of infection, characterized by pneumonia, excessive inflammation, and acute respiratory distress. Finally, the fourth phase is the recovery phase, which addresses diminished lung function, digestion, and fatigue.

Each phase has room for differential diagnosis. TCM practitioners respect the ever-changing nature of viral illnesses and know when to modify or change a formula following the diagnosis at the time of intake. This approach allows TCM practitioners to stay in sync with the patient's health status. As such, the most accurate formulas will match the stage of infection and include modifications per patient.

PHASE 1: IMPROVE HOST DEFENSES

The goal of this phase is to improve the host defense against infection. In TCM diagnostics, this includes nourishing the Zheng Qi (upright energy) and the Wei Qi (protective energy) with herbs and diet. These terms refer to the forms of Qi (energy) that protect the body from external pathogens. In TCM, teaching patients self-care methods, especially those at risk of exposure to viruses, may help decrease the chance of getting infected. Self-care includes decreasing stress, improving sleep, eating, and hydrating well for a balanced immune system. Importantly, practitioners can also teach patients how to improve their nutritional intake and how to support digestive function with nourishing soups and functional foods (see part III below). If patients have any digestive problems or preexisting conditions that need supportive care, this is the phase to address those concerns.

Practitioners can also recommend supportive herbal medicine to improve the host defenses, especially for those with lowered immune function (Wei Qi deficiency) or lymphopenia. Ideally, it is best to educate patients about supportive herbs and foods to have on hand. Proactive self-care, wearing masks, physical distancing, handwashing, appropriate quarantining, and other Covid-19 guidelines may go a long way toward preventing SARS-CoV-2 and other contagious viral respiratory infections.

Phase 1 Herbal Formula 1
1. YU PING FENG SAN – JADE SCREEN POWDER

The main formula for supporting the host immune defense against all viral respiratory infections is *Yu Ping Feng San* (Jade Screen Powder). *Yu Ping Feng San* is a formula from the *Dan Xi Xin Fa* (Dan Xi's Theories) by Zhu Dan Xi in the Yuan Dynasty (1279–1368 CE).

Yu Ping Feng San includes Huang Qi (Astragalus Membranaceus), Bai Zhu (Atractylodis Macrocephalae Rhizome), and Fang Feng (Ledebouriella Divaricata aka Saposhnikoviae Radix or Siler Root). *Yu Ping Feng San* may be particularly useful for patients prone to cold and flu viruses due to lowered immunity (Wei Qi deficiency), e.g., patients with lymphopenia.

Flavonoids, polysaccharides, and saponins from Huang Qi (Astragalus Membranaceus) enhance toll-like receptor expression; increase cytokines, T and B lymphocyte production, natural killer cells, and macrophages (Li et al., 2019; Yin et al., 2010; Shi et al., 2014). Bai Zhu (Atractylodis Macrocephalae

Rhizome) contains the sesquiterpene lactone, atractylon, responsible for its potent antiviral activity (Cheng et al., 2016). Sesquiterpene lactones are a large class of polyphenolic compounds (in food and plants) with various pharmacological activities such as anti-inflammatory, antimicrobial, antioxidant, and antiviral effects (Ozcelik et al., 2009). Fang Feng (Ledebouriella Divaricata) contains chromones, coumarins, lignans, polyacetylenes, and sterols and possesses analgesic, anti-proliferative, antioxidant, and iNOS inhibitory activities (Chin et al., 2011).

Notably, *Yu Ping Feng San* has been shown to induce antiviral protein gene expression and suppress neuraminidase activity of influenza A in cultured epithelial cells, which prevents viral release and spreading (Du et al., 2015). Below is a list of the herbal ingredients and dosages of *Yu Ping Feng San*.

Yu Ping Feng San - Ingredients and Dosages
• Huang Qi (Astragalus Membranaceus) 15g
• Bai Zhu (Atractylodis Macrocephalae Rhizome) 10g
• Fang Feng (Ledebouriella Divaricata) 10g

Preparation and dosage: It is best to soak herbs in 400 ml of water for 20 minutes before cooking. Bring the herbs up to a rolling boil and then lower to a simmer for 20-30 minutes. Each formula is to be taken warm in 2 divided doses between meals in the morning and evening.

The following chart describes the many bioactive compounds and their actions in *Yu Ping Feng San*. Please note studies for each herb referenced in the chart below.

Yu Ping Feng San Ingredients, Bioactive Compounds, and Actions		
Yu Ping Feng San Ingredients	Herb Name	Bioactive Compounds and Actions
	Huang Qi (Astragalus Membranaceus)	Flavonoids: Kaempferol, luteolin, quercetin, apigenin, rutin, daidzein. (Bratkov et al., 2016). Flavonoids, polysaccharides, and saponins from Huang Qi (Astragalus Membranaceus) enhance toll-like receptor expression; increase cytokines, T and B lymphocyte production, natural killer cells, and macrophages (Li et al., 2019; Yin et al., 2010; Shi et al., 2014).
	Fang Feng (Ledebouriella Divaricata)	Flavonoids: Rutin, ferulate (Kim et al., 2018). Fang Feng (Ledebouriella Divaricata) contains chromones, coumarins, lignans, polyacetylenes, and sterols and possesses analgesic,

		antiproliferative, antioxidant, and iNOS inhibitory activities (Chin et al., 2011).
	Bai Zhu (Atractylodis Macrocephalae Rhizome)	Phenolic acids: caffeic acid, ferulic acid, and protocatechuic acid (Li et al., 2012). Contains the antiviral sesquiterpene lactone, atractylon (Cheng et al., 2016).

Autoimmune Disease Caveat

It is important to remember that herbs such as Huang Qi (Astragalus Membranaceus), Echinacea (Echinacea Purpurea), Ren Shen (Radix Ginseng), and Chuan Xin Lian (Andrographis Paniculata), increase immune cells that may already get overexpressed in autoimmune disease patients. Therefore do not use these specific herbs for patients with Multiple Sclerosis, Systemic Lupus Erythematosus, and Rheumatoid Arthritis, et al. autoimmune diseases.

Phase 1 Herbal Formula 2

2. SANG JU YIN – MULBERRY LEAF AND CHRYSANTHEMUM DECOCTION

Sang Ju Yin is a formula from Wu Tang's Qing Dynasty (1368–1911 CE) text, *Wen Bing Tiao Bian* (Systematic Differentiation of Warm Diseases), published in 1798. *Sang Ju Yin* has traditionally been used for upper respiratory infections, including the common cold, influenza, and acute bronchitis (Chen & Hsu).

Sang Ye (Folium Mori) and Flos Chrysanthemi (Ju Hua) are the chief ingredients in *Sang Ju Yin*. Sang Ye (Folium Mori) contains quercetin and kaempferol (flavonols, both known for their antiviral effects), and Chrysanthemum (Ju Hua) contains luteolin. Luteolin is an antiviral flavone that is also known to suppress NFKB production of the inflammatory cytokines TNF-α and IL-6 (Kang et al., 2010), i.e., the precise inflammatory cytokines that overexpress in respiratory distress syndromes, including, Covid-19.

Sang Ju Yin can also be considered for cough, mild fever, and thirst in the early stage of viral infections, including SARS-CoV-2. The goal is to start using the herbs immediately in the early stage of respiratory infections to interrupt the progression from cough to dyspnea to ARDS. Practitioners can also modify *Sang Ju Yin* with Huang Qin (Radix Scutellariae) and Da Qing Ye (Folium Isatidis) to increase the antiviral effects (Chen, 2020).

Modified Sang Ju Yin - Ingredients and Dosages	
• Sang Ye (Folium Mori) 12g • Ju Hua (Flos Chrysanthemi) 10g • Ku Xing Ren (Semen Armeniacae Amarum) 10g • Jie Geng (Radix Platycodi) 10g • Huang Qin (Radix Scutellariae) 9g • Da Qing Ye (Folium Isatidis) 9g	• Lu Gen (Rhizoma Phragmitis) 15g • Lian Qiao (Fructus Forsythiae) 15g • Bo He (Herba Menthae) 6g • Gan Cao (Radix Glycyrrhizae) 6g

Note: It is important to remember that Ku Xing Ren (Semen Armeniacae Amarum) is a tree nut, and should be avoided for patients who have tree nut allergies.

Preparation and dosage: It is best to soak herbs in 400 ml of water for 20 minutes before cooking. Bring the herbs up to a rolling boil and then lower to a simmer for 20-30 minutes. Each formula is to be taken warm in 2 divided doses between meals in the morning and evening.

The following chart describes the many bioactive compounds and their actions in *Sang Ju Yin*. Please note studies for each herb referenced in the chart below.

Sang Ju Yin Ingredients, Bioactive Compounds, and Actions		
Herb in Sang Ju Yin	Herb Name	Bioactive Compounds and Actions
	Sang Ye (Folium Mori)	Flavonoids: Rutin, isoquercitrin, astragalin, kaempferol, quercetin, chlorogenic acid (Zhang et al., 2017). Quercetin, kaempferol, rutin, morin (Chen et al., 2018). Rutin, isoquercitrin, astragalin, gallic acid (Kim et al., 2014). Sang Ye (Folium Mori) could act on the novel coronavirus S-protein binding site of ACE2 (Niu et al., 2020). Contains flavonoids including moralbanone, which has antiviral activity against HSV-1 (Du et al., 2003) and morin, which has anti-asthmathic, anti-COPD, and anti-allergic effects (Middleton et al., 1992).

	Ju Hua (Flos Chrysanthemi)	Apigenin, luteolin, quercetin, hesperetin, hesperidin (Du et al., 2015). Ameliorates acute lung injury via downregulating TLR4/NFKB (Li et al., 2015).
	Bo He (Herba Menthae)	Quercetin, apigenin, hesperetin, hesperidin (Zhu, 1998). Diosmin downregulates the expression of T cell receptors, proinflammatory cytokines and NFKB activation against LPS-induced acute lung injury in mice (Imam et al., 2015).
	Lian Qiao (Fructus Forsythiae)	Luteolin, quercetin, kaempferol, rutin, baicalin, wogonin. Lignans (forsythin) triterpenoids (betulinic acid, oleanolic acid, ursolic acid) (Dong et al., 2017). Forsythoside A has antiviral effects against influenza (Law et al., 2017). Lian Qiao (Fructus Forsythiae) could act on the S-protein binding site of ACE2 to block viral entry of

		SARS-CoV-2 (Niu et al., 2020; Chan et al., 2020).
	Jie Geng (Radix Platycodi)	The saponin, platycodin D, attenuates acute lung injury by suppressing apoptosis and inflammation in vivo and in vitro (Tao et al., 2015). Platycodin D demonstrated high binding affinity to PL^{pro} (Wu et al., 2020).
	Ku Xing Ren (Semen Armeniacae Amarum)	Amygdalin inhibits NFKB and NLRP3 signaling pathways in LPS-induced acute lung injury (Zhang et al., 2017). Amygdalin has an antitussive effect (Miyagoshi et al., 1986).
	Lu Gen (Rhizoma Phragmitis)	Phenolic acids Lignans (Choi et al., 2014).
	Huang Qin (Scutellaria Baicalensis)	Flavonoids Baicalin, chrysin, wogonin, and oroxylin A have therapeutic efficacy against acute lung injury caused by influenza A (H1N1) virus (Zhi et al., 2019).

		Baicalin may bind to the ACE2 enzyme to block entry of SARS-CoV-2 (Chen & Du, 2020).

Chrysin may inhibit 3CL^{pro} and baicalin may inhibit PL^{pro} (Wu et al., 2020).

Scutellarein inhibits the helicase protein in SARS-CoV-1 (Yu et al., 2012).

Scutellarin is predicted to bind to the ACE2 receptor to prevent SARS-CoV-2 entry (Chen & Du, 2020).

Scutellarin suppresses NLP3 inflammasome activation in macrophages, decreases NFKB, IL-6, TNF-α, and IL-1β (Liu et al., 2018; Wang et al., 2016; Tan et al., 2016).

Scutellarin also protects against LPS induced acute lung injury via inhibition of NFKB activation in mice (Tan et al., 2009). |

	Da Qing Ye (Folium Isatidis)	Sinigrin, β-sitosterol, and indigo dose-dependently inhibited cleavage activities of the 3CL^{pro} (Lin et al., 2015).
	Gan Cao (Radix Glycyrrhizae)	Glycyrrhiza Glabra contains the antiviral triterpenoid saponin, glycyrrhizin, found to inhibit SARS-CoV-1 (Cinatl et al., 2003). Glycyrrhizin is predicted to bind to the ACE2 receptor to prevent SARS-CoV-2 entry (Chen & Du, 2020). Glycyrrhizin inhibits IL-6 in macrophages (Liu et al., 2014). Isoliquiritigenin inhibits NFKB activation to suppress the inflammatory response in ARDS (Lago et al., 2014).

Essential Herbs for Essential Workers

The most recommended formula to shore up Wei Qi (protective energy) is *Yu Ping Feng San* (Jade Screen Powder). Some TCM practitioners are also using Huang Qi (Astragalus Membranaceus), plus a combination of Jin Yin Hua (Flos Lonicerae Japonicae), Lian Qiao (Fructus Forsythiae), Mian Ma Guan Zhong (Dryopteris Crassirhizoma), Da Qing Ye (Folium Isatidis), Huang Qin

(Scutellaria Baicalensis), Qing Pi (Pericarpium Citri Reticulate Viride), Huo-Xiang (Herba Agastaches Pogostemonis), Pei Lan (Herba Eupatorii), Cang Zhu (Atractylodes Lancea), and Cao Guo (Fructus Amomi Tsaoko) depending on the presentation (Chen & Hsu, 2020). All of these herbs can also be used to modify *Yu Ping Feng San*. Practitioners who have a loose herb pharmacy or granule extracts can create a unique formula based on the case presentation.

Interestingly, in 2005, Lau et al. showed that a combination of *Sang Ju Yin* (Mulberry Leaf and Chrysanthemum Decoction) and *Yu Ping Feng San* (Jade Windscreen Powder) plus Da Qing Ye (Folium Isatidis) and Huang Qin (Radix Scutellariae) taken for two weeks, helped to prevent viral infections of SARS-CoV-1 in hospital workers compared to those who did not take it.

This combination may be especially helpful for those working on the front lines of healthcare and for every essential worker until we have trusted antiviral treatments or a vaccine. It may also be useful for elderly patients, immune-compromised patients, and concerned patients who are venturing outside more - even with their masks on. For patients and those who might get exposed to others in our workplace or elsewhere, this combination of herbs may help support the protective energy (Wei Qi).

PHASE 2: THE EARLY STAGE OF INFECTION

For all viral respiratory illnesses, if patients present with a pattern of symptoms including sore throat, dry cough, fatigue, myalgia, and digestive upset, make sure they are under the supervision of a medical doctor and have the proper tests done. In TCM diagnostics, the initial signs and symptoms of viral infections (from the common cold to influenza and Covid-19) can present as either 'toxic heat attacking the lung' or 'wind-cold invading the exterior' (the surface of the body). Because the symptoms are slightly different, wind-cold invading the exterior requires a different herbal formulation than toxic heat attacking the lung.

Both toxic heat attacking the lung and wind-cold invading the exterior can cause symptoms of fever, aversion to cold, chills, headache, and myalgia. However, wind-cold presentations usually include muscle stiffness in the neck and back, diarrhea, mild fever without sweating (or no fever at all), and a ticklish sensation in the throat but no dry cough, as may be the case for toxic heat attacking the lung (see below). The practitioner may also observe that the patient's tongue is pale with a thin white coating, and their pulse is floating, which indicates that the body is fighting a pathogen at the exterior level (Chen, 2020). In this case, practitioners who have raw herbs or granule extracts can use a modified version of the *Shang Han Lun* (On Cold Damage) formula *Ge Gen Tang* (Puerariae Decoction).

Phase 2: Wind-Cold Invading the Exterior Formula 1
1. GE GEN TANG – KUDZU DECOCTION

Ge Gen Tang acts to expel wind and release the exterior via diaphoretic and pain-relieving effects. The inclusion of Jin Yin Hua (Flos Lonicerae Japonicae) adds to the formula's antiviral effects. The chart below lists the ingredients and dosages for Modified *Ge Gen Tang*.

Modified Ge Gen Taneg - Ingredients and Dosages	
• Ge Gen (Radix Puerariae Lobatae) 15g	• Zhi Gan Cao (Radix Glycyrrhizae) 10g
• Ma Huang (Herba Ephedrae) 10g	
• Gui Zhi (Ramulus Cinnamomi) 6g	• Bai Shao (Radix Paeoniae Alba) 15g
• Sheng Jiang (Rhizoma Zingiberis Recens) 10g	
• Jin Yin Hua (Flos Lonicerae Japonicae) 20g	• Da Zao (Zizyphus Jujubae) 10g

Preparation and dosage: It is best to soak herbs in 400 ml of water for 20 minutes before cooking. Bring the herbs up to a rolling boil and then lower to a simmer for 20-30 minutes. Each formula is to be taken warm in 2 divided doses between meals in the morning and evening.

The following chart describes the many bioactive compounds and their actions in modified *Ge Gen Tang*. Please note studies for each herb referenced in the chart below.

Modified Ge Gen Tang Ingredients, Bioactive Compounds, and Actions		
Herbs in Modified Ge Gen Tang	Herb Name	Bioactive Compounds and Actions
	Ge Gen (Radix Puerariae Lobatae)	For enhancement of immunity, puerarin, an isoflavonoid from Puerariae Lobatae, increased IFN-γ (Wang et al., 2018).
	Ma Huang (Herba Ephedrae)	Contains quercetin, luteolin, kaempferol, naringin, and β-sitosterol, which all help decrease NFKB and cytokines such as tumor necrosis factor alpha (TNF-α) and IL6, SELE, IL-2 and CXCL10 in asthma (Huang et al., 2020).
	Gui Zhi (Ramulus Cinnamomi)	Cinnamaldehyde inhibits PGE2, IL-1β, tumor necrosis factor-α (TNF-α), and the activation of NFKB for anti-inflammatory effects (Chao et al., 2008; Reddy et al., 2004).

	Bai Shao (Radix Paeoniae Alba)	Paeonol from Paeonia Lactiflora shows antiviral activity against rhinovirus (Ngan et al., 2015).
	Sheng Jiang (Rhizoma Zingiberis Recens)	Gingerol, allicin, and shogaol (Eng et al., 2019). Allicin in ginger (Zingiber officinale) inhibits influenza A (H1N1) (neuraminidase (Sahoo et al., 2016).
	Zhi Gan Cao (Radix Glycyrrhizae)	Glycyrrhiza Glabra contains the antiviral triterpenoid saponin, glycyrrhizin, found to inhibit SARS-CoV-1 (Cinatl et al., 2003). Glycyrrhizin is predicted to bind to the ACE2 receptor to prevent SARS-CoV-2 entry (Chen & Du, 2020). Glycyrrhizin inhibits IL-6 in macrophages (Liu et al., 2014). Isoliquiritigenin inhibits NFKB activation to suppress the inflammatory response in ARDS (Lago et al., 2014).

	Da Zao (Zizyphus Jujubae)	Oleanolic acid, betulinic acid, quercetin, apigenin (Eng et al., 2019).
	Jin Yin Hua (Flos Lonicerae Japonicae)	Luteolin, kaempferol, quercetin, apigenin, rutin, caffeic acid, chlorogenic acid, lonicerin (Xu et al., 2019). Chlorogenic acid in Flos Lonicerae Japonicae has antiviral activity against influenza A (H1N1/H3N2) and inhibition of neuraminidase (Ding et al., 2017). Homosecoiridoid alkaloids in Flos Lonicerae Japonicae have antiviral activity against the influenza virus H3N2 (Yu et al., 2013). Flos Lonicerae Japonicae could act on the S-protein binding site of ACE2 to block viral entry of SARS-CoV-2 (Niu et al., 2020; Chan et al., 2020).

Further Modifications of Ge Gen Tang

Xiang Ru (Herba Moslae) 3-10g can be used as a substitute for Ma Huang (Herba Ephedrae). For headache add Bai Zhi (Radix Angelicae Dahuricae) 15g, and for a ticklish sensation in the throat, add She Gan (Rhizoma Belamcandae) 15g (Chen, 2020).

Phase 2: Wind-Cold Invading the Exterior Formula 2

2. CHAI GE JIE JI TANG - BUPLEURUM AND PUERARIA COMBINATION

Another herbal formula for wind-cold symptoms of fever and chills, headache, and stiffness in the upper extremities, is *Chai Ge Jie Ji Tang* (Bupleurum and Pueraria Combination to Release the Muscle Layer). *Chai Ge Jie Ji Tang* is a formula from the 15th-century medical source text, *Shang Han Lui Shu* (Six Texts of Cold Induced Disorders). Below is a list of the herbal ingredients and dosages for *Chai Ge Jie Ji Tang*.

Chai Ge Jie Ji Tang - Ingredients and Dosages	
• Chai Hu (Radix Bupleuri) 9g	• Bai Shao (Radix Paeoniae Alba) 9g
• Ge Gen (Radix Puerariae Lobatae) 15g	• Jie Geng (Radix Platycodi) 9g
• Shi Gao (Gypsum Fibrosum) 15-30g (pre-decoct)	• Sheng Jiang (Rhizoma Zingiberis Recens) 6g
• Qiang Huo (Rz/Rx Notopterygii) 10g	• Da Zao (Fructus Jujubae) 6g
• Bai Zhi (Radix Angelicae Dahuricae) 9g	• Gan Cao (Radix Glycyrrhizae) 6g
• Huang Qin (Radix Scutellariae) 9g	

Preparation and dosage: Note the dosage of Shi Gao (Gypsum) can be adjusted based on the severity of fever (Chen & Hsu, 2020). It is best to soak herbs in 400 ml of water for 20 minutes before cooking. Bring the herbs up to a rolling boil and then lower to a simmer for 20-30 minutes. Each formula is to be taken warm in 2 divided doses between meals in the morning and evening.

The following chart describes the many bioactive compounds and their actions in *Chai Ge Jie Ji Tang*. Please note studies for each herb referenced in the chart below.

Chai Ge Jie Ji Tang Ingredients, Bioactive Compounds, and Actions		
Herbs in Chai Ge Jie Ji Tang	Herb Name	Bioactive Compounds and Actions
	Ge Gen (Radix Puerariae Lobatae)	For enhancement of immunity, puerarin, an isoflavonoid from Puerariae Lobatae, increased IFN-γ (Wang et al., 2018).
	Bai Zhi (Angelicae Dahuricae Radix)	Anti-nociceptive and anti-inflammatory effects of Angelicae Dahuricae Radix through inhibition of the expression of inducible nitric oxide synthase and NO production (Kang et al., 2008).
	Chai Hu (Radix Bupleuri)	Contains saikosaponin B2, which exerts antiviral activity against human coronaviruses (Cheng et al., 2006).

	Bai Shao (Radix Paeoniae Alba)	Paeonol from Paeonia lactiflora shows antiviral activity against rhinovirus (Ngan et al., 2015).
	Sheng Jiang (Rhizoma Zingiberis Recens)	Gingerol, allicin, and shogaol (Eng et al., 2019). Allicin in ginger (Zingiber officinale) inhibits influenza A (H1N1) neuraminidase (Sahoo et al., 2016).
	Gan Cao (Radix Glycyrrhizae)	Glycyrrhiza Glabra contains the antiviral triterpenoid saponin, glycyrrhizin, found to inhibit SARS-CoV-1 (Cinatl et al., 2003). Glycyrrhizin is predicted to bind to the ACE2 receptor to prevent SARS-CoV-2 entry (Chen & Du, 2020). Glycyrrhizin inhibits IL-6 in macrophages (Liu et al., 2014). Isoliquiritigenin inhibits NFKB activation to suppress the inflammatory response in ARDS (Lago et al., 2014).

	Da Zao (Zizyphus Jujubae)	Oleanolic acid, betulinic acid, quercetin, apigenin (Eng et al., 2019).
	Jie Geng (Radix Platycodi)	Platycodin D attenuates acute lung injury by suppressing apoptosis and inflammation in vivo and in vitro (Tao et al., 2015). Platycodin D demonstrated high binding affinity to PL^{pro} (Wu et al., 2020)
	Huang Qin (Scutellaria Baicalensis)	Baicalin, chrysin wogonin, and oroxylin A have therapeutic efficacy against acute lung injury caused by influenza A (H1N1) virus (Zhi et al., 2019). Baicalin may bind to the ACE2 enzyme to block entry of SARS-CoV-2 (Chen & Du, 2020). Chrysin may inhibit 3CL^{pro} and baicalin may inhibit PL^{pro} (Wu et al., 2020).

		Scutellarein inhibits the helicase protein in SARS-CoV-1 (Yu et al., 2012).
	Shi Gao (Gypsum Fibrosum)	Gypsum CaSO4·2H2O Gypsum compounds have anti-inflammatory and antipyretic effects decreasing the PGE2 level in the hypothalamus (Zhou et al., 2012).
	Qiang Huo (Rhizoma and Radix Notopterygii)	Improves dysfunctional metabolomics in influenza A (H1N1) pneumonia (Chen et al., 2014).

PHASE 2: FORMULA FOR WIND-COLD INVASION WITH INTERNAL DAMPNESS

HUO XIANG ZHENG QI WAN - AGASTACHE FORMULA TO RECTIFY THE QI

Huo Xiang Zheng Qi Wan is a formula from the *Tai Ping Hui Min He Ji Ju Fang* (Imperial Grace Formulary of the Tai Ping Era) written in 1078 CE during the Song Dynasty (960–1279 CE) by the Taiping Huimin Pharmaceutical Bureau (Traditional Medicine Research, 2020). *Huo Xiang*

Zheng Qi Wan has traditionally been used for a pattern of wind-cold invasion with internal dampness, which presents as headache, fever, myalgia, nausea, vomiting, abdominal pain, and diarrhea.

Since gastrointestinal symptoms may precede sore throat and dyspnea, e.g., in the case of Covid-19, *Huo Xiang Zheng Qi Wan* can be considered for digestive support. For example, *Huo Xiang Zheng Qi Wan* can be used if signs and symptoms include headache, fever, myalgia, nausea, vomiting, abdominal pain, and diarrhea. If patients only have GI distress, myalgia, and fever without a sore throat, dry cough, or dyspnea, this still may indicate that the virus is in the body but not yet attacking the lungs. At this point, practitioners might consider combining *Yin Qiao San* (see below) along with *Huo Xiang Zheng Qi Wan*. Practitioners can use raw herbs, granule extracts, or the pill form for each formula.

Huo Xiang Zheng Qi Wan - Ingredients and Dosages	
• Huo Xiang (Herba Agastaches Pogostemonis) 15g	• Bai Zhu (Atractylodis Macrocephalae Rhizome) 12g
• Gan Cao (Radix Radix Glycyrrhizae) 12g	• Fu Ling (Sclerotium Poriae Cocos) 12g
• Jie Geng (Radix Platycodi) 10g	• Zi Su Ye (Folium Perillae) 12g
• Hou Po (Cortex Magnoliae Officinalis) 12g	• Bai Zhi Radix (Angelicae Dahuricae) 9g
• Zhi Ban Xia (Rhizoma Pinelliae Preparata) 12g	• Da Fu Pi (Pericarpium Arecae Catechu) 12g
• Chen Pi (Pericarpium Citri Reticulatae) 12g	• Da Zao (Zizyphus Jujubae) 6g

Preparation and dosage: It is best to soak herbs in 400 ml of water for 20 minutes before cooking. Bring the herbs up to a rolling boil and then lower to a simmer for 20-30 minutes. Each formula is to be taken warm in 2 divided doses between meals in the morning and evening.

The following chart describes the many bioactive compounds and their actions in *Huo Xiang Zheng Qi Wan*. Please note studies for each herb referenced in the chart below.

Huo Xiang Zheng Qi Wan Ingredients, Bioactive Compounds, and Actions		
Huo Xiang Zheng Qi Wan Ingredients	Herb Name	Bioactive Compounds and Actions
	Huo Xiang (Herba Agastaches Pogostemonis)	Phenylpropanoids, terpenoids, phenolics, rosmarinic acid, agastachin (Zielińska, & Matkowski, 2014). Patchouli alcohol contained in Guang Huo Xiang (Herba Pogostemonis) inhibits 3CL^{pro} and, therefore, viral replication of SARS-CoV-2 (Wu et al., 2020). Patchouli alcohol in Guang Huo Xiang (Herba Pogostemonis) also acts on the ACE2 receptor to prevent viral entry (Wu et al., 2020). Contains pachypodol, a tri-O-methyl ether of quercetin that inhibits

		several human pathogenic RNA viruses, including rhinovirus, coxsackievirus and poliovirus, acting on viral plus-strand RNA replication (Ishitsuka et al., 1982).
	Gan Cao (Radix Glycyrrhizae)	Glycyrrhiza Glabra contains the antiviral triterpenoid saponin, glycyrrhizin, found to inhibit SARS-CoV-1 (Cinatl et al., 2003). Glycyrrhizin is predicted to bind to the ACE2 receptor to prevent SARS-CoV-2 entry (Chen & Du, 2020). Glycyrrhizin inhibits IL-6 in macrophages (Liu et al., 2014). Isoliquiritigenin inhibits NFKB activation to suppress the inflammatory response in ARDS (Lago et al., 2014).

| | Jie Geng (Radix Platycodi) | Platycodin D attenuates acute lung injury by suppressing apoptosis and inflammation in vivo and in vitro (Tao et al., 2015).

Platycodin D demonstrated high binding affinity to PL^{pro} (Wu et al., 2020). |
|---|---|---|
| | Hou Po (Cortex Magnoliae Officinalis) | Quercetin, kaempferol Magnolol, honokiol (Rajgopal et al., 2016).

Aporphine alkaloids were shown to interfere with the viral replicative cycle of poliovirus (Boustie et al., 1998). |
| | Zhi Ban Xia (Rhizoma Pinelliae Preparata) | Baicalein, β-sitosterol, shogaol, and gingerol inhibit NFKB in acute airway viral infections (Eng et al., 2019). |
| | Chen Pi (Pericarpium Citri Reticulatae) | Nobiletin ameliorates inflammation in acute lung injury by suppression of NFKB pathway in vivo and vitro (Li et al., 2018).

Hesperetin from Pericarpium Citri |

		Reticulatae is predicted to bind with ACE2 (Chen & Du, 2020).
	Bai Zhu (Atractylodis Macrocephalae Rhizome)	Phenolic acids: caffeic acid, ferulic acid, and protocatechuic acid (Li et al., 2012). Contains the antiviral sesquiterpene lactone, atractylon (Cheng et al., 2016).
	Fu Ling (Sclerotium Poriae Cocos)	Poria Cocos Polysaccharide (PCP) has immunomodulatory activity through TLR4, TRAF6, and NFKB signaling both in vitro and in vivo (Tian et al., 2019).
	Bai Zhi (Angelicae Dahuricae Radix)	Anti-nociceptive and anti-inflammatory effects of Angelicae Dahuricae Radix through inhibition of inducible nitric oxide synthase and NO production (Kang et al., 2008).
	Da Fu Pi (Pericarpium Arecae Catechu)	Areca catechu plant extracts inhibited syncytium formation, and trafficking of the hemagglutinin-neuraminidase (HN) glycoprotein to the cell-surface in Newcastle

		disease virus (NDV) (Lee et al., 2014).
	Zi Su Ye (Folium Perillae)	Anthocyanins, rosmarinic acid.

Anti-allergic, anti-inflammatory, antioxidant, anticancer, antimicrobial, antidepressant, and anti-cough effects (Yu et al., 2017). |
| | Da Zao (Zizyphus Jujubae) | Oleanolic acid, betulinic acid, quercetin, apigenin (Eng et al., 2019). |

Toxic Heat Attacking the Lung

In TCM diagnostics, if toxic heat is attacking the lung, patients will likely present with symptoms of fever, aversion to cold, sore throat, dry cough, scanty sputum, myalgia, fatigue, and headache. The tip and sides of the tongue may be red, and the tongue may appear to have a thin white or thin yellow coating. In this pattern, the pulse will likely be floating and rapid (Chen, 2020). In TCM, practitioners can select herbs to clear heat and detoxify poisons, i.e., to inhibit the virus and stop it from replicating. Keep in mind that many 'clear heat' herbs offer a three-hit effect acting as antivirals that lead to NFKB inhibition and, therefore, reduce cytokine production and inflammation.

Phase 2: Toxic Heat Attacking the Lung Formula 1
1. *YIN QIAO SAN* - HONEYSUCKLE AND FORSYTHIA POWDER

Several formulas that address 'toxic heat attacking the lung' may be used for this pattern. The first formula, *Yin Qiao San* (Honeysuckle and Forsythia Powder), also comes from Wu Tang's *Wen Bing Tiao Bian* (Systematic Differentiation of Warm Diseases), published in 1798. *Yin Qiao San* can be considered as supportive therapy for symptoms of sore throat, slight chills, fever, dry cough, aversion to wind, and mild or no sweating in the early stages of upper respiratory infections.

Yin Qiao San - Ingredients and Dosages	
• Jin Yin Hua (Flos Lonicerae Japonicae) 10g	• Dan Zhu Ye (Herba Lophatheri) 10g
• Lian Qiao (Fructus Forsythiae) 10g	• Lu Gen (Rhizoma Phragmitis) 15g
• Jing Jie (Herba Schizonepetae) 10g	• Gan Cao (Radix Glycyrrhizae) 10g
• Niu Bang Zi (Fructus Arctii) 10g	• Jie Geng (Radix Platycodi) 10g
• Bo He (Herba Menthae) 10g	
• Dan Dou Chi (Semen Sojae Praeparatum) 10g	

Note: It is important to remember that this formula contains Dan Dou Chi (Semen Sojae Praeparatum) soybeans, and should be avoided for patients who have soy allergies.

Preparation and dosage: It is best to soak herbs in 400 ml of water for 20 minutes before cooking. Bring the herbs up to a rolling boil and then lower to a simmer for 20-30 minutes. Each formula is to be taken warm in 2 divided doses between meals in the morning and evening.

The following chart describes the many bioactive compounds and their actions in *Yin Qiao San*. Please note studies for each herb referenced in the chart below.

Yin Qiao San Ingredients, Bioactive Compounds, and Actions		
Herbs in Yin Qiao San	Herb Name	Bioactive Compounds

		and Actions
	Jin Yin Hua (Flos Lonicerae Japonicae)	Luteolin, kaempferol, quercetin, apigenin, rutin, caffeic acid, chlorogenic acid, lonicerin (Xu et al., 2019). Chlorogenic acid in Flos Lonicerae Japonicae has antiviral activity against influenza A (H1N1/H3N2) and inhibition of neuraminidase (Ding et al., 2017). Homosecoiridoid alkaloids in Flos Lonicerae Japonicae have antiviral activity against the influenza virus H3N2 (Yu et al., 2013). Flos Lonicerae Japonicae could act on the S-protein binding site of ACE2 to block viral entry of SARS-CoV-2 (Niu et al., 2020; Chan et al., 2020).

	Lian Qiao (Fructus Forsythiae)	Luteolin, quercetin, kaempferol, rutin, baicalin, wogonin. Lignans (forsythin) triterpenoids (betulinic acid, oleanolic acid, ursolic acid) (Dong et al., 2017). Forsythoside A has antiviral effects against influenza (Law et al., 2017). Fructus Forsythiae could act on the S-protein binding site of ACE2 to block viral entry of SARS-CoV-2 (Niu et al., 2020; Chan et al., 2020).
	Lu Gen (Rhizoma Phragmitis)	Phenolic acids Lignans (Choi et al., 2014).

	Dan Dou Chi (Semen Sojae Praeparatum)	Isoflavone daidzein has been reported to inhibit the protease activity of SARS-CoV-1 3CL^{pro} (Jo et al., 2020). Nicotianamine is a novel ACE2 inhibitor in soybean (Takahashi et al., 2015).
	Niu Bang Zi (Fructus Arctii)	Arctigenin attenuates acute lung injury (Shi et al., 2015).
	Jing Jie (Herba Schizonepetae)	Schizonepetin, a monoterpene from Herba Schizonepetae, is a potential antiviral agent (Geng et al., 2011).
	Jie Geng (Radix Platycodi)	Platycodin D attenuates acute lung injury by suppressing apoptosis and inflammation in vivo and in vitro (Tao et al., 2015). Platycodin D demonstrated high binding affinity to PL^{pro} (Wu et al., 2020)

	Herba Menthae (Bo He)	Quercetin, apigenin, hesperetin, hesperidin (Zhu, 1998). Diosmin downregulates the expression of T cell receptors, proinflammatory cytokines and NFKB activation against LPS-induced acute lung injury in mice (Imam et al., 2015).
	Dan Zhu Ye (Herba Lophatheri)	Luteolin, apigenin, chlorogenic acid (Ma et al., 2020). Herba Lophatheri possesses antiviral, anti-bacterial, anti-cancer, antioxidant, diuretic, and hyperglycemic properties (Kim et al., 2016).
	Gan Cao (Radix Glycyrrhizae)	Glycyrrhiza Glabra contains the antiviral triterpenoid saponin, glycyrrhizin, found to inhibit SARS-CoV-1 (Cinatl et al., 2003). Glycyrrhizin is predicted to bind to the ACE2 receptor to prevent SARS-CoV-2 entry (Chen & Du, 2020).

		Glycyrrhizin inhibits IL-6 in macrophages (Liu et al., 2014). Isoliquiritigenin inhibits NFKB activation to suppress the inflammatory response in ARDS (Lago et al., 2014).

Practitioners can also modify the above formulas with the following herbs.

Additional Antiviral Herb Options	
• Huang Qin (Scutellaria Baicalensis) • Ban Lan Gen (Radix Isatidis) • Da Qing Ye (Folium Isatidis) • Pu Gong Ying (Herba Taraxaci) • Ye Ju Hua (Flos Chrysanthemi Indici) • Sang Ye (Folium Mori) • Qing Hao (Artemisia Annua)	• Huang Lian (Rhizoma Coptidis) • Zi Hua Di Ding (Herba Violae) • Yu Xing Cao (Houttuynia Cordata) • Huo Xiang (Herba Agastaches Pogostemonis)

For a strong cough in the early stage of infection, the following herbs can be added to either *Sang Ju Yin* or *Yin Qiao San*.

Additional Options for Cough in the Early Stage of Respiratory Infections
• Sang Bai Pi (Morus Alba Bark) • Pi Pa Ye (Folium Eriobotryae) • Zi Su Ye (Folium Perillae)

Phase 2: Toxic Heat Attacking the Lung Formula 2
2. LIAN HUA QING WEN CAPSULE

Lian Hua Qing Wen Capsule is a Chinese herbal product that is recommended for patients that present with mild initial symptoms of fatigue and fever in Covid-19 (The People's Republic of China National Health Commission, 2020). Notably, *Lian Hua Qing Wen Capsule* has shown in vitro inhibition of various influenza viruses (Ding et al., 2017). The compounds in *Lian Hua Qing Wen Capsule* have also been shown to block the early stages of influenza virus infection and to inhibit virus-induced gene expression of IL-6, IL-8, TNF-α, IP-10, and MCP-1 (ibid, 2017). Because these cytokines and chemokines are elevated in acute respiratory distress presentations, the compounds in *Lian Hua Qing Wen Capsule* may help quiet this increased immune activity in Covid-19.

A study by Dong et al. (2014) reported that the levels of IL-8, TNF-α, IL-17, and IL-23 in the sputum and of IL-8 and IL-17 in the blood of patients who had an acute exacerbation of chronic obstructive pulmonary disease (COPD), markedly decreased after treatment with *Lian Hua Qing Wen Capsules*. Most remarkably, this formula was recently studied for SARS-CoV-2 in vitro and did better than the viral polymerase inhibitor Remdesivir by significantly inhibiting SARS-CoV-2 replication in Vero E6 cells and markedly reducing proinflammatory cytokines (TNF-α, IL-6, CCL-2/MCP-1, and CXCL-10/IP-10) production at the mRNA levels (Li et al., 2020).

An analysis of *Lian Hua Qing Wen Capsules* revealed that quercetin, luteolin, kaempferol, rutin, naringenin, β-sitosterol, wogonin, lonicerin, aloe-emodin, 18β-glycyrrhetinic acid, indigo, forsythoside, hyperoside, salidroside, and other compounds are in this formula (Huang et al., 2020).

Lian Hua Qing Wen Capsule Ingredients:

- Lian Qiao (Fructus Forsythiae)
- Jin Yin Hua (Flos Lonicerae Japonicae)
- Xing Ren (Semen Armeniacae Amarum)
- Shi Gao (Gypsum Fibrosum)
- Ban Lan Gen (Isatis Indigotica)
- Guan Zhong (Dryopteris Crassirhizoma)
- Ma Huang (Ephedra Sinica)
- Bo He Nao (Mentha Haplocalyx)
- Yu Xing Cao (Houttuynia Cordata)
- Huo Xiang (Herba Agastaches Pogostemonis)
- Da Huang (Rheum Palmatum)
- Hong Jing Tian (Rhodiola Rosea)
- Gan Cao (Radix Glycyrrhizae)

The following chart describes the many bioactive compounds and their actions in *Lian Hua Qing Wen Capsules*. Please note studies for each herb referenced in the chart below.

Lian Hua Qing Wen Capsule Ingredients, Bioactive Compounds, and Actions		
Lian Hua Qing Wen Ingredients	Herb Name	Bioactive Compounds and Actions

	Jin Yin Hua (Flos Lonicerae Japonicae)	Luteolin, kaempferol, quercetin, apigenin, rutin, caffeic acid, chlorogenic acid, lonicerin (Xu et al., 2019). Chlorogenic acid in Flos Lonicerae Japonicae has antiviral activity against influenza A (H1N1/H3N2) and inhibition of neuraminidase (Ding et al., 2017). Homosecoiridoid alkaloids in Flos Lonicerae Japonicae have antiviral activity against the influenza virus H3N2 (Yu et al., 2013). Flos Lonicerae Japonicae could act on the S-protein binding site of the ACE2 receptor to block viral entry of SARS-CoV-2 (Niu et al., 2020; Chan et al., 2020).

| | Lian Qiao (Fructus Forsythiae) | Luteolin, quercetin, kaempferol, rutin, baicalin, wogonin.

Lignans (forsythin) triterpenoids (betulinic acid, oleanolic acid, ursolic acid) (Dong et al., 2017).

Forsythoside A has antiviral effects against influenza (Law et al., 2017).

Fructus Forsythiae could act on the S-protein binding site of ACE2 to block viral entry of SARS-CoV-2 (Niu et al., 2020; Chan et al., 2020). |
|---|---|---|
| | Xing Ren (Semen Armeniacae Amarum) | Amygdalin inhibits NFKB and NLRP3 signaling pathways in LPS-induced acute lung injury (Zhang et al., 2017).

Amygdalin has an antitussive effect (Miyagoshi et al., 1986). |
| | Hong Jing Tian (Radix et Rhizoma Rhodiola Crenulata) | Proanthocyanidins, rosavin, salidroside (Chiang et al., 2015).

Kaempferol, epicatechin, quercetin, catechin, naringenin, luteolin, p-coumaric acid, ellagic acid, ferulic acid, epigallocatechin, |

			chlorogenic acid, epicatechin gallate, and epigallocatechin gallate (Lewicki et al., 2017).
	Bo He Nao (Mentha haplocalyx)		Quercetin, apigenin, hesperetin, hesperidin (Zhu, 1998). Diosmin downregulates the expression of T cell receptors, proinflammatory cytokines and NFKB activation against LPS-induced acute lung injury in mice (Imam et al., 2015).
	Yu Xing Cao (Houttuynia Cordata)		Quercetin, quercetrin, cinanserin (Chiow et al., 2016). Plant polysaccharides from Houttuynia Cordata (Yu Xing Cao) were shown to reduce pulmonary edema, protein exudation, and the deposition of complement activation products, thereby mitigating acute lung injury in rats (Lu et al., 2018). Houttuynia Cordata (Yu Xing Cao) blocked viral RNA-dependent RNA

		polymerase activity of SARS-CoV-1 (Lau et al., 2008). Quercetin, quercetrin, and cinanserin from the water extract of Houttuynia Cordata (Yu Xing Cao) blocked SARS-CoV-1 3CL^{pro} (Lau et al., 2008).
	Ban Lan Gen (Isatis Indigotica)	Sinigrin, β-sitosterol, and indigo dose-dependently inhibited cleavage activities of the 3CL^{pro} (Lin et al., 2015). Phaitanthrin D and 2,2-di (3-indolyl)-3-indolone from Isatis Indigotica (Ban Lan Gen) may inhibit PL^{pro} (Wu et al., 2020).
	Shi Gao (Gypsum Fibrosum)	Gypsum CaSO4·2H2O Gypsum compounds have anti-inflammatory and antipyretic effects decreasing the PGE2 level in the hypothalamus (Zhou et al., 2012).

	Gan Cao (Radix Glycyrrhizae)	Glycyrrhiza Glabra contains the antiviral triterpenoid saponin, glycyrrhizin, found to inhibit SARS-CoV-1 (Cinatl et al., 2003). Glycyrrhizin is predicted to bind to the ACE2 receptor to prevent SARS-CoV-2 entry (Chen & Du, 2020). Glycyrrhizin inhibits IL-6 in macrophages (Liu et al., 2014). Isoliquiritigenin inhibits NFKB activation to suppress the inflammatory response in ARDS (Lago et al., 2014).
	Da Huang (Rheum Palmatum)	Emodin from genus Rheum Palmatum (Da Huang) blocks 3CL^{pro} (Luo et al., 2009) and markedly inhibited the interaction of SARS-CoV-1 S-protein and ACE2 (Ho et al., 2007). Emodin inhibits the 3a (viral) ion channel of SARS-CoV-1 and may potentially prevent viral release from infected cells (Schwarz et

		Huo Xiang (Giant Hyssop, Agastaches)	al., 2011; Schwarz et al., 2014).
			Phenylpropanoids, terpenoids, phenolics, rosmarinic acid, agastachin (Zielińska, & Matkowski, 2014).
			Patchouli alcohol contained in Guang Huo Xiang (Herba Pogostemonis) inhibits 3CL^{pro} and, therefore, viral replication of SARS-CoV-2 (Wu et al., 2020).
			Patchouli alcohol in Guang Huo Xiang (Herba Pogostemonis) also acts on the ACE2 receptor to prevent viral entry (Wu et al., 2020).
			Contains pachypodol, a tri-O-methyl ether of quercetin that inhibits several human pathogenic RNA viruses, including rhinovirus, coxsackievirus and poliovirus, acting on viral plus-strand RNA replication (Ishitsuka et al., 1982).

	Ma Huang (Ephedra Sinica)	Inhibits PGE2 biosynthesis, reduces IgE-mediated histamine release, reduces the mRNA or protein levels of IL-1β, IL-6, TNF-α, COX2, and NFKB (Zhang et al., 2018).
	Mian Ma Guan Zhong (Dryopteris Crassirhizoma)	Mian Ma Guan Zhong contains kaempferol, which blocks PL^{pro} and 3CL^{pro}, and has the potential to inhibit SARS-CoV-2 (Zhang et al., 2020).

While *Lian Hua Qing Wen Capsules* contain Ma Huang (Ephedra Sinica), which is banned in the US and elsewhere, practitioners may be able to reproduce the formula with granule extracts or loose herbs using Xiang Ru (Herba Moslae) 3-10g as a substitute for Ma Huang. Interestingly, a spectral analysis of Herba Moslae (Xiang Ru) revealed many similar flavonoids as Herba Ephedrae (Ma Huang), including luteolin, quercetin, and apigenin (Hu et al., 2010).

Phase 2: Toxic Heat Attacking the Lung Formula 3
3. SHUANG HUANG LIAN

The research on another formula, *Shuang Huang Lian*, is worth considering as another example of the routine use of the same potent compounds for viral and other respiratory infections that produce excessive amounts of cytokines and inflammation. The medicinal herbs in *Shuang Huang Lian*, including Flos Lonicerae Japonicae (Jin Yin Hua), Scutellaria Baicalensis (Huang Qin), and Fructus Forsythiae (Lian Qiao), all have demonstrated antiviral activity against

SARS-CoV-1 as well as for many strains of influenza (Zheng, 2010). This effect is primarily due to the potent combination of antiviral compounds, including chlorogenic acid in Jin Yin Hua (Flos Lonicerae Japonicae), forsythoside A in Lian Qiao (Fructus Forsythiae), and baicalin in Huang Qin (Scutellaria Baicalensis) (Lem et al., 2020).

Shuang Huang Lian has also been shown to markedly reduce the transcriptional and translational levels of inflammatory cytokines TNF-α, IL-1β, and IL-6 in lipopolysaccharide-stimulated murine alveolar macrophages (Gao et al., 2014). Because these are the precise cytokines that get overexpressed in response to SARS-CoV-2, all of these herbs may help quiet this overzealous immune activity that comes with Covid-19.

The bioactive ingredients in *Shuang Huang Lian* were also shown to attenuate airway hyperresponsiveness and inflammation in a murine asthma model (Gao et al., 2019). The herbs in *Shuang Huang Lian* can be taken in pill form, granule extracts, or prepared as a decoction. While *Shuang Huang Lian*, like all of the herb formulas in this book, has not yet been tested in clinical trials to prove its efficacy against SARS-CoV-2, we can still appreciate the potent antiviral effects of each of these herbs, especially when used synergistically in herbal formulas for viral respiratory infections.

The following chart describes the many bioactive compounds and their actions in *Shuang Huang Lian*. Please note studies for each herb referenced in the chart below.

Shuang Huang Lian Ingredients, Bioactive Compounds, and Actions		
Shuang Huang Lian Ingredients	Bioactive Compounds and Actions	Formulas for Covid-19

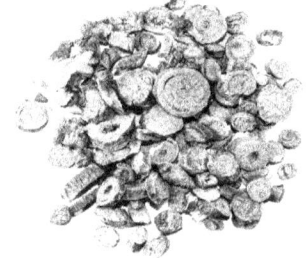	Huang Qin (Scutellaria Baicalensis)

Baicalin, chrysin, wogonin, and oroxylin A have therapeutic efficacy against acute lung injury caused by influenza A virus (H1N1) (Zhi et al., 2019).

Baicalin may bind to the ACE2 enzyme to block entry of SARS-CoV-2 (Chen & Du, 2020).

Chrysin may inhibit 3CL^{pro} and baicalin may inhibit PL^{pro} (Wu et al., 2020).

Scutellarein inhibits the helicase protein in SARS-CoV-1 (Yu et al., 2012).

Scutellarin is predicted to bind to the ACE2 receptor to prevent SARS-CoV-2 entry (Chen & Du, 2020).

Scutellarin suppresses NLP3 inflammasome activation in macrophages, decreases NFKB, IL-6, TNF-α, and IL-1β (Liu et al., 2018; Wang et al., 2016; Tan et al., 2016). | *Shuang Huang Lian*

Qing Fei Pai Du Tang

Chai Ge Jie Ji Tang

Modified Yu Ping Feng San |

	Scutellarin also protects against LPS induced acute lung injury via inhibition of NFKB activation in mice (Tan et al., 2009).	
	Lian Qiao (Fructus Forsythiae) Luteolin, quercetin, kaempferol, rutin, baicalin, wogonin. Lignans (forsythin) triterpenoids (betulinic acid, oleanolic acid, ursolic acid) (Dong et al., 2017). Forsythoside A has antiviral effects against influenza (Law et al., 2017). Fructus Forsythiae could act on the S-protein binding site of ACE2 to block viral entry of SARS-CoV-2 (Niu et al., 2020; Chan et al., 2020).	*Shuang Huang Lian* *Yin Qiao San* *Lian Hua Qing Wen Capsule* *Modified Yu Ping Feng San*

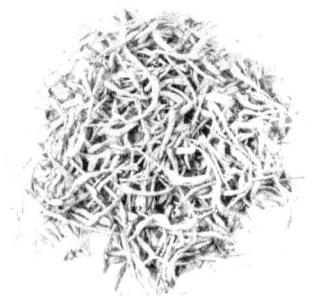	Jin Yin Hua (Flos Lonicerae Japonicae) Luteolin, kaempferol, quercetin, apigenin, rutin, caffeic acid, chlorogenic acid, lonicerin (Xu et al., 2019). Chlorogenic acid in Flos Lonicerae Japonicae has antiviral activity against influenza A (H1N1/H3N2) and inhibition of neuraminidase (Ding et al., 2017). Homosecoiridoid alkaloids in Flos Lonicerae Japonicae have antiviral activity against the influenza virus H3N2 (Yu et al., 2013). Flos Lonicerae Japonicae could act on the S-protein binding site of ACE2 to block viral entry of SARS-CoV-2 (Niu et al., 2020; Chan et al., 2020).	*Shuang Huang Lian* *Yin Qiao San* *Lian Hua Qing Wen Capsule* *Modified Yu Ping Feng San*

Phase 2: Early Stage of Infection with High Fever
BAI HU TANG – WHITE TIGER DECOCTION

Bai Hu Tang is another formula from the *Shang Han Lun* (On Cold Damage) that has traditionally been used for high fever, profuse sweating, severe thirst, and a large pulse, which indicates that the body is fighting a pathogenic factor. The following chart includes the ingredients and dosages for *Bai Hu Tang*. White Tiger Decoction can be added to *Yin Qiao San* and *San Ju Yin* for a stronger effect in the initial stage of infection, especially if there is a high fever (Chen, 2020).

Bai Hu Tang- Ingredients and Dosages	
• Gypsum Fibrosum (Shi Gao) 15-30g (pre-decoct) • Anemarrhena Rhizome (Zhi Mu) 15g	• Sweet Rice (Nuo Mi) 30g • Radix Glycyrrhizae (Gan Cao) 6g

PHASE 3: ACUTE LUNG INVOLVEMENT AND PNEUMONIA

Most practitioners will likely only see patients with mild to moderate lung symptoms, as most Covid-19 pneumonia and acute respiratory distress cases will need emergency and intensive care. At this stage, the CT scan will likely reveal both lungs to have multiple scattered or large pieces of ground-glass opacity (GGO) (Chen & Hsu, 2020). At this stage, from a TCM perspective, the viral invasion has progressed from the exterior to the interior resulting in damp-heat and toxic stagnation obstructing the lung. In this pattern, signs and symptoms may include fever, chills, cough, dyspnea, and chest oppression. The tongue may appear pale with a greasy white coating, and the pulse may be soft or slippery (ibid, 2020).

If the patient is not hospitalized and is already under the supervision of a medical doctor, supportive herbal therapy with a formula based on *Qing Fei Pai Du Tang* (see below) may be helpful.

Phase 3: Acute Lung Involvement - Pneumonia Formula

QING FEI PAI DU TANG – CLEAR THE LUNG AND ELIMINATE TOXINS DECOCTION

Qing Fei Pai Du Tang is the premier formula used in China for mild to acute respiratory symptoms, including pneumonia and severe acute respiratory distress cases that are simultaneously treated with western medications and interventions. In the United States, practitioners will likely not have access to hospitalized or critically ill patients where treatment interventions such as ventilators will be necessary. For patients who need extra support for mild to moderate respiratory symptoms, including pneumonia, *Qing Fei Pai Du Tang* contains a potent combination of herbs that may help decrease the severity of the infection, modulate the immune system, reduce inflammation, and support respiratory function. Other formulas that *Qing Fei Pai Du Tang* is based on, such as *Ma Xing Shi Gan Tang*, can also be considered for pneumonia (see historical antecedents of *Qing Fei Pai Du Tang* below).

Below are the twenty-one herbs in *Qing Fei Pai Du Tang* that are recommended in China for Covid-19 patients (People's Republic of China National Health Commission; Chen & Hsu, 2020). Please note additional studies for each herb referenced in the chart below.

Qing Fei Pai Du Tang - Ingredients and Dosages	
<ul><li>Ma Huang (Herba Ephedrae) 9g</li><li>Zhi Gan Cao (Radix et Rhizoma Glycyrrhizae Praeparata cum Melle) 6g</li><li>Ku Xing Ren (Semen Armeniacae Amarum) 9g</li><li>Shi Gao (Gypsum Fibrosum) 15-30g (pre-decoct)</li><li>Gui Zhi (Ramulus Cinnamomi) 9g</li><li>Ze Xie (Rhizoma Alismatis) 9g</li><li>Zhu Ling (Polyporus) 9g</li><li>Bai Zhu (Rhizoma Atractylodis Macrocephalae 9g</li><li>Fu Ling (Sclerotium Poriae Cocos) 15g</li><li>Chai Hu (Radix Bupleuri) 16g</li><li>Huang Qin (Radix Scutellariae) 6g</li><li>Jiang Ban Xia (Rhizoma Pinelliae Praeparatum cum Zingiber) 9g</li></ul>	<ul><li>Sheng Jiang (Rhizoma Zingiberis Recens) 9g</li><li>Zi Wan (Radix et Rhizoma Asteris) 9g</li><li>Kuan Dong Hua (Flos Farfarae) 9g</li><li>She Gan (Rhizoma Belamcandae) 9g</li><li>Xi Xin (Radix et Rhizoma Asari) 6g</li><li>Shan Yao (Rhizoma Dioscoreae) 12g</li><li>Zhi Shi (Fructus Aurantii Immaturus) 6g</li><li>Chen Pi (Pericarpium Citri Reticulatae) 6g</li><li>Guang Huo Xiang (Herba Pogostemonis) 9g</li></ul>

Please note that because Kuan Dong Hua (Flos Farfarae) contains senkirkine and senecionine, which are potentially hepatotoxic and carcinogenic pyrrolizidine alkaloids, it must be used with extreme caution for patients with pre-existing liver disorders (Neuman et al., 2015). Instead of Kuan Dong Hua (Flos Farfarae), practitioners can substitute Pi Pa Ye (Folium Eriobotryae) 6g (Chen, 2020). Zi Wan (Radix et Rhizoma Asteris) can also be hepatotoxic with extended use and should only be used for short periods in general and not at all for patients who have liver problems (Peng et al., 2016).

Preparation and dosage: Note the dosage of Shi Gao (Gypsum) can be adjusted based on the severity of fever (Chen & Hsu, 2020). It is best to soak herbs in 400 ml of water for 20 minutes before cooking. Bring the herbs up to a rolling boil and then lower to a simmer for 20-30 minutes.

Each formula is to be taken warm in 2 divided doses between meals in the morning and evening.

The following chart describes the many bioactive compounds and their actions in *Qing Fei Pai Du Tang*. Please note additional studies for each herb in the chart below.

Qing Fei Pai Du Tang Ingredients, Bioactive Compounds, and Actions		
Herbs in Qing Fei Pai Du Tang	Herb Name	Bioactive Compounds and Actions
	Shi Gao (Gypsum FIbrosum)	Gypsum $CaSO_4 \cdot 2H_2O$ Gypsum has an antipyretic effect by decreasing the PGE2 level in the hypothalamus (Zhou et al., 2012).
	Zhi Shi (Fructus Aurantii Immaturus)	Hesperidin, neohesperidin, hesperetin, rutin, rhoifolin, naringenin (Bai et al., 2018). Hesperidin and neohesperidin demonstrate potential as M^{pro} inhibitors (Khaerunnisa et al., 2020). Hesperetin is predicted to

		bind to the ACE2 receptor to prevent SARS-CoV-2 entry (Chen & Du, 2020).
		Hesperidin has high binding affinity to the helicase protein in SARS-CoV-2 (Wu et al., 2020).
		Hesperidin ameliorates acute lung injury (ALI) by inhibiting HMGB1 release (Liu et al., 2015).
		Naringin has a protective effect against ALI (Fouad et al., 2016).
	Ma Huang (Ephedra Stem)	Contains quercetin, luteolin, kaempferol, naringenin, and β-sitosterol which all help decrease NFKB and cytokines such as tumor necrosis factor alpha (TNF-α) and IL6, SELE, IL-2 and CXCL10 in asthma (Huang et al., 2020).
		Ephedrannin A and B, from Ephedra Sinica, effectively suppressed the transcription of TNF-α, IL-1β, and NFKB, and the phosphorylation of p38 mitogen-activated protein (MAP) kinase to exert their anti-inflammatory actions on

		LPS-stimulated macrophages (Kim et al., 2010).
	Huo Xiang (Giant hyssop aerial part)	Phenylpropanoids, terpenoids, phenolics, rosmarinic acid, agastachin (Zielińska, & Matkowski, 2014). Contains pachypodol, a tri-O-methyl ether of quercetin that inhibits several human pathogenic RNA viruses, including rhinovirus, coxsackievirus and poliovirus, acting on viral plus-strand RNA replication (Ishitsuka et al., 1982).
	Ku Xing Ren (Semen Armeniacae Amarum)	Amygdalin inhibits NFKB and NLRP3 signaling pathways in LPS-induced acute lung injury (Zhang et al., 2017). Amygdalin has an antitussive effect (Miyagoshi et al., 1986).
	Chai Hu (Radix Bupleuri)	Contains saikosaponin B2, which exerts antiviral activity against human coronaviruses (Cheng et al., 2006).

	Chen Pi (Pericarpium Citri Reticulatae)	Nobiletin ameliorates inflammation in acute lung injury by suppression of NFKB pathway in vivo and vitro (Li et al., 2018). Hesperetin from Pericarpium Citri Reticulatae is predicted to bind with ACE2 (Chen & Du, 2020).
	Gui Zhi (Cassia twig)	Procyanidin from Cinnamomum Cassia may effectively inhibit the replication of the influenza virus (Dai et al., 2012). Coumarin in Cinnamomum Cassia inhibits influenza A (H1N1) neuraminidase (Sahoo et al., 2016).
	Zhi Gan Cao (Radix Glycyrrhizae)	Glycyrrhiza Glabra contains the antiviral triterpenoid saponin, glycyrrhizin, found to inhibit SARS-CoV-1 (Cinatl et al., 2003). Glycyrrhizin is predicted to bind to the ACE2 receptor to prevent SARS-CoV-2 entry (Chen & Du, 2020). Glycyrrhizin inhibits IL-6 in macrophages (Liu et al., 2014). Isoliquiritigenin inhibits NFKB activation to suppress

			the inflammatory response in ARDS (Lago et al., 2014).
		Jiang Ban Xia (Rhizoma Pinelliae Praeparatum cum Zingiber)	Baicalein, β-sitosterol, shogaol, and gingerol inhibit NFKB in acute airway viral infections (Eng et al., 2019).
		Bai Zhu (Atractylodis Macrocephalae Rhizome)	Phenolic acids: caffeic acid, ferulic acid, and protocatechuic acid (Li et al., 2012). Contains the antiviral sesquiterpene lactone, atractylon (Cheng et al., 2016).
		Zhu Ling (Polyporus Umbellatus)	Polyporus Umbellatus Polysaccharide (PUPS) has been identified as the major bioactive component in the mushroom Polyporus Umbellatus that has immuno-enhancing, anti-tumor, anti-inflammatory, and hepatoprotective activities (Guo et al., 2019). Polyporus Umbellatus polysaccharide has inhibitory effect on hepatitis B (Liu et al., 2001).

	Fu Ling (Sclerotium Poriae Cocos)	Poria Cocos Polysaccharide (PCP) has immunomodulatory activity through TLR4, TRAF6, and NFKB signaling both in vitro and in vivo (Tian et al., 2019).
	She Gan (Rhizoma Belamcandae)	Flavonoids, terpenoids, quinones, iristectogenin A, genistein, belamcandin, luteolin, phenolic compounds, gallic acid, isoferulic acid, ursolic acid (Zhang et al., 2016). Irigenin, a major active constituent of Rhizoma Belamcandae, can reduce NO and PGE2 production by decreasing the mRNA and protein expression of iNOS and COX-2, respectively, as well as by suppressing NFKB activation in murine macrophages (Ahn et al., 2006).
	Xi Xin (Radix et Rhizoma Asari)	Asatone inhibits NFKB and MAPK signaling pathways to prevent acute lung injury in vitro (Chang et al., 2018).

	Sheng Jiang (Rhizoma Zingiberis Recens)	Gingerol, shogaol, and allicin (Eng et al., 2019).

Allicin in ginger (Zingiber officinale) inhibits influenza A (H1N1) neuraminidase (Sahoo et al., 2016). |
| | Zi Wan (Radix et Rhizoma Asteris) | Asterosaponins, chlorogenic acid (Zhao et al., 2014). Quercetin (Zhou et al., 2004).

Aster Tataricus can protect from LPS-induced acute lung injury mainly through inhibiting the release of inflammatory cells (WBC, macrophage, neutrophil, lymphocyte), regulating the proinflammatory cytokines (IL-1β, IL-6, TNF-α), and attenuating pulmonary edema (Chen et al., 2019).

Monoterpene glycosides in Aster Tataricus suppressed NO production, inflammatory cytokines (prostaglandin E2, interleukin-6, and interleukin-1 beta) and the expression of inflammatory enzymes (inducible nitric oxide synthase and cyclooxygenase-2) via inhibition of NFKB |

		activation, and prevented the downstream activation of the p38 mitogen-activated protein kinase (MAPK) pathways by inhibiting phosphorylation of c-Jun N-terminal kinases, and extracellular signal-regulated kinases (Su et al., 2019).
	Pi Pa Ye (Eriobotrya Japonica) Pi Pa Ye is a substitute for Kuan Dong Hua (Flos Farfarae)	Quercetin, kaempferol (Luoati et al., 2003). Triterpenes in Eriobotrya Japonica have antifibrotic effects in pulmonary fibrosis (Yang et al., 2012).
	Shan Yao (Dioscorea rhizome)	Dioscin alleviates acute lung injury through suppression of TLR4 signaling pathways (Jun et al., 2018).
	Scutellaria Baicalensis (Huang Qin)	Baicalein, chrysin, wogonin, and oroxylin A have therapeutic efficacy against acute lung injury caused by influenza A (H1N1) virus (Zhi et al., 2019). Baicalin may bind to the ACE2 enzyme to block entry of SARS-CoV-2 (Chen & Du, 2020). Chrysin may inhibit 3CL^{pro} and baicalin may inhibit

		PL^{pro} (Wu et al., 2020). Scutellarein inhibits the helicase protein in SARS-CoV-1 (Yu et al., 2012). Scutellarin is predicted to bind to the ACE2 receptor to prevent SARS-CoV-2 entry (Chen & Du, 2020). Scutellarin suppresses NLP3 inflammasome activation in macrophages, decreases NFKB, IL-6, TNF-α, and IL-1β (Liu et al., 2018; Wang et al., 2016; Tan et al., 2016). Scutellarin also protects against LPS induced acute lung injury via inhibition of NFKB activation in mice (Tan et al., 2009).
	Ze Xie (Rhizoma Alismatis)	Triterpenoids, alisols et al. sesquiterpenoids and diterpenoids posess diuretic, antimetabolic disorder, hepatoprotective, immunomodulatory, antiosteoporotic, anti-inflammatory, antitumor, and antibacterial activities) (Zhang et al., 2017).

Analysis of Qing Fei Pai Du Tang

The herbs in *Qing Fei Pai Du Tang* (Clear the Lung and Eliminate Toxins Decoction) have multiple therapeutic properties including, antiviral, antipyretic, immune-modulating, and anti-inflammatory effects. When used for Covid-19, the compounds in *Qing Fei Pai Du Tang* may help to reduce fever (with antiviral and antipyretic herbs), relieve cough and phlegm (with antitussive herbs), drain dampness (with diuretic herbs), balance the immune system, and decrease inflammation (i.e., with immune-modulating and anti-inflammatory herbs). A recent observational study revealed that 41.8% of 214 Covid-19 pneumonia cases in China developed ARDS (Wu et al., 2020; National Administration of Traditional Chinese Medicine, 2020). This same study reported that *Qing Fei Pai Du Tang* was effective among 90% of cases and that 60% of patients had improved radiological findings with limited detail (ibid, 2020).

Based on the reported beneficial results of faster recovery times and decreased severity of other symptoms such as fatigue, poor appetite, and sore throat, *Qing Fei Pai Du Tang* was officially recommended for Covid-19 by the National Health Commission of the People's Republic of China and National Administration of Traditional Chinese Medicine. Given this information, it seems that interrupting the progression of pneumonia into ARDS may potentially help to decrease the mortality rate of Covid-19.

Since inflammatory responses by the immune system to the virus contribute to the death of patients with Covid-19, it may be possible that immune-modulating and anti-inflammatory agents help reduce the severity of the immune and inflammatory responses and the mortality rate for patients. Acute lung injury (ALI) characterized by pulmonary edema and diffuse alveolar damage (DAD) can cause acute progressive respiratory distress and persistent hypoxemia (Ding et al., 2020). Acute respiratory distress syndrome (ARDS) is a severe progression of ALI and a possible outcome of Covid-19. It is not surprising that many of these same herbs used for ALI and ARDS have found their way into *Qing Fei Pai Du Tang* and other formulas for Covid-19 patients. A recent network pharmacology analysis demonstrated that *Qing Fei Pai Du Tang* regulates key immunological pathways (Th17 cell differentiation, T cell, and B cell signaling) and TNF signaling pathways (Zhao et al., 2020; Chan et al., 2020).

Attenuating the Cytokine Storm and Decreasing Inflammation

SARS-CoV-1 and SARS-CoV-2 infections and resultant acute respiratory distress lead to the activation of NFKB and a cascade of inflammatory molecules such as IFN-gamma, CXCL10, IL-18, IL-10, IL-1β, TNF-α, and IL-6, MCP-1, IL-8 and p38 mitogen-activated protein kinase (MAPK) pathways which can lead to an increase of TGFβ and IL-2 (Zhang et al., 2018; Huang et al., 2020). The 'cytokine storm' that occurs in severe cases of Covid-19 is a prolonged overactive immune-inflammatory response that often affects elderly and immune-compromised individuals or those with other pre-existing conditions. During the cytokine storm, an excessive amount of immune activity in response to the virus can trigger immune-mediated pulmonary damage and inflammation as the immune system continues to try to eliminate the infection. Severe acute respiratory distress syndrome, diffuse alveolar damage, respiratory failure, and fibrosis can also occur due to both the virus and the immune system's response to it.

The cytokine storm causes an upregulation of inflammasome NLRP3 via caspase-1 proteases, which results in NFKB activation, IL-1β, IL-18 production, and cell death (Yun & Yi, 2019). In this case, herbs that have immune-modulating properties may help decrease NFKB, IL-1β, IL-18, TNF-α, IL-6, et al. upregulated chemical messengers while also inhibiting the virus and reducing inflammation. Antiviral herbs that are high in kaempferol, quercetin, luteolin, saponins, and saikosaponins can reduce lung inflammation and balance the immune system via decreasing NFKB and cytokine production et al. upregulated chemokines.

For example, Herba Ephedrae (Ma Huang) contains five potent compounds, including quercetin, luteolin, kaempferol, naringenin, and β-sitosterol, which all help decrease NFKB and cytokines such as tumor necrosis factor-alpha (TNF-α) and IL6 (ibid, 2015). Quercetin and luteolin have also been shown to decrease SELE, IL-2, and CXCL10 at protein and mRNA levels, which may explain why Ma Huang (Herba Ephedrae) is so effective against inflammation in asthma (Huang et al., 2020). Ephedrine in Ma Huang also directly activates alpha- and beta-adrenergic receptors to reduce bronchial mucosal edema and to dilate the bronchus, respectively (Miyagoshi et al., 1986; Abourashed et al., 2003). For added respiratory support, Ku Xing Ren (Semen Armeniacae Amarum) contributes antitussive amygdalin, which also inhibits NFKB and NLRP3 signaling pathways in LPS-induced acute lung injury (Miyagoshi et al., 1986; Zhang et al., 2017).

Asatone in Xi Xin (Radix et Rhizoma Asari) helps prevent acute lung injury by reducing expressions of NFKB, MAPK, and inflammatory cytokines (Chang et al., 2018). Baicalin et al. flavonoids derived from Huang Qin (Scutellaria Baicalensis), glycyrrhizin from Gan Cao (Radix Glycyrrhizae), saikosaponin B from Chai Hu (Radix Bupleuri), allicin and gingerols from Sheng Jiang (Rhizoma Zingiberis Recens), along with other bioactive compounds, contribute to the overall antiviral, immune-modulating, and anti-inflammatory effects of this formula. Please refer to the chart of *Qing Fei Pai Du Tang* to further consider the combined therapeutic effect of all the herb compounds in this formula.

Availability of Qing Fei Pai Du Tang

If you practice in the United States, this formula is not yet fully available. The reason *Qing Fei Pai Du Tang* can't be reproduced here is that three of the ingredients are banned by the U.S. Food & Drug Administration (FDA), i.e., Herba Ephedrae (Ma Huang) and Radix et Rhizoma Asari (Xi Xin) and Kuan Dong Hua (Flos Farfarae). Yet, if needed, most of the herbs in *Qing Fei Pai Du Tang* can likely be sourced in the form of loose herbs or single herb granule extracts with substitutions for Ma Huang (Herba Ephedrae), Xi Xin (Radix et Rhizoma Asari) and Kuan Dong Hua (Flos Farfarae). For example, Xiang Ru (Herba Moslae) 3-10g can be used as a substitute for Ma Huang, Gan Jiang (Rhizoma Zingiberis) 6g can be used instead of Xi Xin (Radix et Rhizoma Asari, and Pi Pa Ye (Eriobotrya Japonica) 6g can be used as a substitute for Kuan Dong Hua (Flos Farfarae (Chen, 2020).

While there are still no randomized controlled trials on *Qing Fei Pai Du Tang* for SARS-CoV-2, we can study the active compounds in this formula that may lead to these effects. Importantly, John Chen, Ph.D., OMD, L.Ac., who is an authority on Chinese medicine and Pharmacology, is working with medical doctors at UCLA, UCSD, and UCI to get FDA approval for the use of Ma Huang (Herba Ephedrae), Xi Xin (Radix et Rhizoma Asari) and Kuan Dong Hua (Flos Farfarae). If approved, their team will be able to carry out a three-arm study of *Qing Fei Pai Du Tang* for Covid-19 patients. In this study, one arm will get a placebo, one arm will get a mushroom supplement, and the other arm will get *Qing Fei Pai Du Tang* (Chen, 2020). Considering the already well-researched effect of many of the same compounds on SARS-CoV-1, ALI, and ARDS, traditional Chinese herbs show promise for pneumonia in Covid-19.

HISTORICAL ANTECEDENTS OF QING FEI PAI DU TANG

Qing Fei Pai Du Tang contains 21 herbal ingredients comprising the following four classical remedies that aim to decrease the severity of symptoms and speed recovery. Because many of the herbs in each of these formulas are featured in *Qing Fei Pai Du Tang*, let's review how the following formulas have been used historically for other viral respiratory illnesses and how that might be similarly applied today.

1. *Ma Xing Shi Gan Tang*
2. *She Gan Ma Huang Tang*
3. *Xiao Chai Hu Tang*
4. *Wu Ling San*

1. MA XING SHI GAN TANG - DECOCTION OF EPHEDRA, APRICOT KERNEL, GYPSUM, AND LICORICE

Ma Xing Shi Gan Tang, a formula from the *Shang Han Lun* (On Cold Damage) by Zhang Jong Jing, has been used historically for an attack of wind-heat on the lung or wind-cold, which has turned into heat with fever, (with or without sweating), cough, shortness of breath, and thirst (Chen, 2020). In terms of biomedical symptomatology, *Ma Xing Shi Gan Tang* is often used for pneumonia, asthma, pertussis, and bronchitis (Kao et al., 2001).

Ma Xing Shi Gan Tang Ingredients	
• Ma Huang (Herba Ephedrae) • Xing Ren (Semen Armeniacae Amarum)	• Zhi Gan Cao (Radix Glycyrrhizae Preparata) • Shi Gao (Gypsum Fibrosum)

The herbs in *Ma Xing Shi Gan Tang* can be likened to a cocktail of bioactive ingredients. These ingredients include ephedrine for bronchodilation, antitussive amygdalin, antiviral glycyrrhizin, and antipyretic gypsum. Research on *Ma Xing Shi Gan Tang* shows that its anti-inflammatory effects are related to regulation of complement cascades, thrombin, and Toll-Like Receptor (TLR) signaling pathways in a rat model of LPS-induced pneumonia (Yang et al., 2020). *Ma Xing Shi Gan Tang* was also found to dampen the progression of pulmonary fibrosis, which is commonly seen in ARDS (Fei et al., 2019). These ingredients and effects may explain its use over many centuries and current inclusion in *Qing Fei Pai Du Tang*, the most recommended formula for pneumonia in Covid-19 patients in China.

2. XIAO CHAI HU TANG - MINOR BUPLEURUM DECOCTION

Xiao Chai Hu Tang is another formula that appears in both the *Shang Han Lun* (On Cold Damage) and the *Jin Gui Yao Lue* (Essential Prescriptions of the Golden Cabinet), the two classical medical treatises compiled by Zhang Zhong Jing during his lifetime (150-219 CE). *Xiao Chai Hu Tang* has been used historically for a bitter taste in the mouth, dry throat, dizziness, alternating chills and fever, fullness in the hypochondrium, fatigue, loss of appetite, and restlessness and is used frequently for many other viral infections (Kong et al., 2018).

Xiao Chai Hu Tang Ingredients	
• Chai Hu (Radix Bupleuri) • Huang Qin (Scutellaria Baicalensis) • Ren Shen (Radix Ginseng) • Ban Xia (Rhizoma Pinelliae) • Da Zao (Zizyphus Jujubae)	• Zhi Gan Cao (Radix Glycyrrhizae Preparata) • Sheng Jiang (Rhizoma Zingiberis Recens)

The herbs in *Xiao Chai Hu Tang* contain a number of bioactive ingredients, including antivirals saikosaponin B2, glycyrrhizin, baicalin, baicalein, scuttelarin, scuttelarein, allicin, gingerols, β-sitosterol, ginsenosides, shogaol, and betulinic acid. All of these ingredients combined inhibit viral infections and decrease inflammation. This potent combination may explain its continued use for viral infections.

3. SHE GAN MA HUANG TANG - BELAMCANDA AND EPHEDRA DECOCTION

Since the ingredients in *She Gan Ma Huang Tang* are also featured heavily in *Qing Fei Pai Du Tang*, let's also review how this formula has been used historically. *She Gan Ma Huang Tang* is another formula from the *Jin Gui Yao Lue* (Essential Prescriptions of the Golden Cabinet).

She Gan Ma Huang Tang has been used historically for deep-seated phlegm in the lungs that lead to wheezing, dyspnea, and asthma (Chen, 2020). *She Gan Ma Huang Tang* can also be used for pulmonary effusion, pulmonary edema, and inflammation in the lungs (Ying, 2020). The chief ingredients of this formula, She Gan (Rhizoma Belamcandae), Ma Huang (Herba Ephedrae), and Ku Xing Ren (Semen Armeniacae Amarum), are included in *Qing Fei Pai Du Tang*. Almost all of the herbs in *She Gan Ma Huang Tang* are included in *Qing Fei Pai Du Tang*. Xiang Ru (Herba Moslae) 3-10g can be used as a substitute for Ma Huang (Herba Ephedrae). *She Gan Ma Huang Tang* can also be used as a recovery formula.

She Gan Ma Huang Tang Ingredients	
• She Gan (Rhizoma Belamcandae) • Zi Wan (Radix et Rhizoma Asteris) • Ma Huang (Herba Ephedrae) • Ban Xia (Rhizoma Pinelliae) • Sheng Jiang (Rhizoma Zingiberis Recens)	• Kuan Dong Hua (Tussilago Flower) • Xi Xin (Radix et Rhizoma Asari) • Hong Zao (Zizyphus Jujubae) • Wu Wei Zi (Schisandra Fruit)

The herbs in *She Gan Ma Huang Tang* contain many bioactive compounds, including ephedrine in Ma Huang, a key ingredient for bronchodilation. Asatone in Xi Xin (Radix et Rhizoma Asari), plus schizandrin and deoxyschizandrin in Wu Wei Zi (Schisandra Fruit) all prevent acute lung injury by reducing expressions of NFKB, MAPK, and inflammatory cytokines, in acute airway viral infections (Chang et al., 2018; Eng et al., 2019).

She Gan Ma Huang Tang also contains the antiviral triterpene, betulinic acid, from Hong Zao (Zizyphus Jujubae), and allicin in ginger (Rhizoma Zingiberis Recens), which inhibits influenza A (H1N1) neuraminidase (Sahoo et al., 2016). Irigenin from the rhizomes of She Gan (Belamcandae Chinensis) has inhibitory effects on nitric oxide and prostaglandinE (2) production in murine macrophages (Ahn et al., 2008). Finally, baicalein, β-sitosterol, shogaol, and gingerol in Ban Xia (Rhizoma Pinelliae) inhibit NFKB in acute airway viral infections (Eng et al., 2019).

4. WU LING SAN – FIVE-INGREDIENT POWDER WITH PORIA

All five of the herbs in *Wu Ling San* are included in *Qing Fei Pai Du Tang*. *Wu Ling San,* mentioned in both the *Shang Han Lun* (On Cold Damage) and *Jin Gui Yao Lue* (Essential Prescriptions of the Golden Cabinet), has traditionally been used for external wind-cold with dampness and phlegm, headache, fever, restlessness, shortness of breath, and acute nephritis, among other presentations. Ze Xie (Rhizoma Alismatis) and Zhu Ling (Polyporus Umbellatus) in this formula have demonstrated diuretic and hepatoprotective effects, respectively (Guo et al., 2019; Zhang et al., 2017).

Wu Ling San Ingredients	
• Zhu Ling (Polyporus Umbellatus) • Ze Xie (Rhizoma Alismatis) • Bai Zhu (Rhizoma Atractylodis Macrocephalae)	• Fu Ling (Poria) • Gui Zhi (Ramulus Cinnamomi)

The herbs in this formula contain many antiviral, anti-inflammatory, diuretic, and hepatoprotective ingredients. Antiviral atractylon in Bai Zhu (Rhizoma Atractylodis Macrocephalae) (Cheng et al., 2016) and Cinnamaldehyde from Gui Zhi (Ramulus Cinnamomi) inhibits PGE2, IL-1β, tumor necrosis factor-α (TNF-α), and the activation of NFKB for anti-inflammatory effects (Chao et al., 2008; Reddy et al., 2004). Zhu Ling (Polyporus Umbellatus) has immuno-enhancing, antitumor, anti-inflammatory, and hepatoprotective effects (Guo et al., 2019). Ze Xie (Rhizoma Alismatis) contains triterpenoids, alisols et al. sesquiterpenoids, and diterpenoids that possess diuretic, antimetabolic disorder, hepatoprotective, immunomodulatory, antiosteoporotic, anti-inflammatory, antitumor, and antibacterial activities) (Zhang et al., 2017).

Now that we have considered the historical antecedents and analyzed *Qing Fei Pai Du Tang* from a more modern perspective, let's review some additional formulas that may help clear excessive phlegm.

ADDITIONAL FORMULAS TO CLEAR EXCESSIVE PHLEGM

1. QING QI HUA TAN WAN - CLEAR THE QI AND TRANSFORM PHLEGM PILL

For deep-seated phlegm, practitioners can use herb formulas such as *She Gan Ma Huang Tang* above or, for excessive phlegm *Qing Qi Hua Tan Wan*, can be used. *Qing Qi Hua Tan* Wan is a formula from the book, *Yi Fang Kao* (Investigations of Medical Formulas) published in 1584 by Wu Kun during the Ming Dynasty (1368–1644 CE). *Qing Qi Hua Tan Wan* has traditionally been used for cough, bronchitis, pneumonia, and emphysema.

Qing Qi Hua Tan Wan - Ingredients and Dosages	
• Zhi Ban Xia (Rhizoma Pinelliae) 9g • Huang Qin (Scutellariae Baicalensis) 15g • Fu Ling (Sclerotium Poriae Cocos) 15g • Zhi Shi (Fructus Aurantii Immaturus) 15g • Dan Nan Xing (Arisaema Bile) 9g	• Ku Xing Ren (Semen Armeniacae Amarum) 15g • Gua Lou (Fructus Trichosanthis) 15g • Chen Pi (Pericarpium Citri Reticulatae) 15g

Preparation and dosage: It is best to soak herbs in 400 ml of water for 20 minutes before cooking. Bring the herbs up to a rolling boil and then lower to a simmer for 20-30 minutes. Each formula is to be taken warm in 2 divided doses between meals in the morning and evening.

Additional Formulas to Clear Excessive Phlegm
2. DING CHUAN TANG - ARREST WHEEZING DECOCTION

Another formula that may be very helpful for excessive phlegm is *Ding Chuan Tang*, which has historically been used for bronchial asthma. *Ding Chuan Tang* is a formula from the book, *Fu Shou Jing Fang* (Exquisite Formulas for Fostering Longevity), written by Wu Min in 1530 CE (Dharmananda, 1997; Bensky & Barolet, 1990).

Ding Chuan Tang may also be useful for clearing excessive phlegm and restoring normal lung function after a viral respiratory illness. In this formula, Xiang Ru (Herba Moslae) can be used as a substitute for Ma Huang (Herba Ephedra), while Pi Pa Ye (Eriobotrya Japonica) 6g can be used as a substitute for Kuan Dong Hua (Flos Farfarae).

Ding Chuan Tang - Ingredients and Dosages	
<ul><li>Ma Huang (Herba Ephedrae) 9g</li><li>Bai Guo (Ginkgo Biloba Seed) 9g</li><li>Sang Bai Pi (Morus Alba Bark) 12g</li><li>Jie Geng (Platycodon Grandiflorum Root) 12g</li><li>Zi Su Zi (Perilla Frutescens Fruit) 9g</li><li>Xing Ren (Prunus Armeniaca Seed) 12g</li><li>Kuan Dong Hua (Flos Farfarae) 6g</li></ul>	<ul><li>Zi Wan (Radix et Rhizoma Asteris) 9g</li><li>Huang Qin (Scutellaria Baicalensis Root) 9g</li><li>Ban Xia (Pinellia Ternata Rhizome) 6g</li><li>Gan Cao (Radix Glycyrrhizae) 6g</li><li>Bai Bu (Stemona tuberosa) 9g</li></ul>

Preparation and dosage: It is best to soak herbs in 400 ml of water for 20 minutes before cooking. Bring the herbs up to a rolling boil and then lower to a simmer for 20-30 minutes. Each formula is to be taken warm in 2 divided doses between meals in the morning and evening.

The following chart describes the many bioactive compounds and their actions in *Ding Chuan Tang*. Please note studies for each herb referenced in the chart below.

Ding Chuan Tang Ingredients, Bioactive Compounds, and Actions		
Herbs in Ding Chuan Tang	Herb Name	Bioactive Compounds and

		Actions
	Bai Guo (Ginkgo Biloba Semen)	Ergosterol peroxide in Ginkgo Biloba (Bai Guo) has antiviral activity (Lindquist et al., 1989). Ginkgo has antitussive and anti-asthmatic effects (Gupta et al., 2010; Jaber, 2002).
	Sang Bai Pi (Morus Alba Bark)	Extracts of Sang Bai Pi (Morus Alba Bark) show antiasthmatic effects via enhancement of CD4 + CD 25 + Foxp3 + regulatory T cells and inhibition of Th2 cytokines in a mouse asthma model (Kim et al., 2011). Morus Alba Bark contains flavonoids, including moralbanone, which has antiviral activity against HSV-1 (Du et al., 2003), and morin, which has anti-asthmatic, anti-COPD, and anti-allergic effects (Middleton et al., 1992).

	Ma Huang (Ephedra Stem)	Contains quercetin, luteolin, kaempferol, naringenin, and β-sitosterol which all help decrease NFKB and cytokines such as tumor necrosis factor alpha (TNF-α) and IL6, SELE, IL-2 and CXCL10 in asthma (Huang et al., 2020). Ephedrannin A and B, from Ephedra Sinica, effectively suppressed the transcription of TNF-α, IL-1β, and NFKB, and the phosphorylation of p38 mitogen-activated protein (MAP) kinase to exert their anti-inflammatory actions on LPS-stimulated macrophages (Kim et al., 2010).
	Bai Bu (Stemona tuberosa)	The main alkaloidal constituents, protostemonine, stemospironine, and maistemonine showed significant antitussive activity (Yang et al., 2008). Stemona tuberosa Has antiviral activity against Dengue virus (Phurimsak & Leardkamolkarn, 2005).

| | Ku Xing Ren (Semen Armeniacae Amarum) | Amygdalin inhibits NFKB and NLRP3 signaling pathways in LPS-induced acute lung injury (Zhang et al., 2017).

Amygdalin has an antitussive effect (Miyagoshi et al., 1986). |
|---|---|---|
| | Zi Su Zi (Perilla Frutescens Fruit) | Contains flavonoids: scutellarein, luteolin, apigenin, and anthocyanins (cis-shisonin and shisonin)

Phenylpropanoids and essential oils perillene, beta-caryophyllene, limonene, and myristicine have antiviral effects (Ahmed, 2019).

Perilla has antitussive effects (Asif, 2012). |
| | Jie Geng (Radix Platycodi) | Saponin, platycodin D, attenuates acute lung injury by suppressing apoptosis and inflammation in vivo and in vitro (Tao et al., 2015).

Platycodin D demonstrated high binding affinity to PL^{pro} (Wu et al., 2020). |

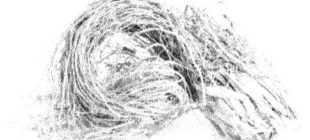	Zi Wan (Radix et Rhizoma Asteris)	Asterosaponins, chlorogenic acid (Zhao et al., 2014). Quercetin (Zhou et al., 2004). Aster Tataricus can protect from LPS-induced acute lung injury mainly through inhibiting the release of inflammatory cells (WBC, macrophage, neutrophil, lymphocyte), regulating the proinflammatory cytokines (IL-1β, IL-6, TNF-α), and attenuating pulmonary edema (Chen et al., 2019). Monoterpene glycosides in Aster Tataricus suppressed NO production, inflammatory cytokines (prostaglandin E2, interleukin-6, and interleukin-1 beta) and the expression of inflammatory enzymes (inducible nitric oxide synthase and cyclooxygenase-2) via inhibition of NFKB activation, and prevented the downstream activation of the p38 mitogen-activated protein kinase (MAPK) pathways by inhibiting phosphorylation of c-Jun N-terminal kinases, and

		extracellular signal-regulated kinases (Su et al., 2019).
	Gan Cao (Radix Glycyrrhizae)	Glycyrrhiza Glabra contains the antiviral triterpenoid saponin, glycyrrhizin, found to inhibit SARS-CoV-1 (Cinatl et al., 2003). Glycyrrhizin is predicted to bind to the ACE2 receptor (Chen & Du, 2020). Glycyrrhizin inhibits IL-6 in macrophages (Liu et al., 2014). Isoliquiritigenin inhibits NFKB activation to suppress the inflammatory response in ARDS (Lago et al., 2014).
	Ban Xia (Pinellia Rhizome)	Baicalein, β-sitosterol, shogaol, and Gingerol inhibit NFKB in acute airway viral infections (Eng et al., 2019).
	Pi Pa Ye (Eriobotrya Japonica) Pi Pa Ye is a substitute for Kuan Dong Hua	Quercetin Kaempferol (Luoati et al., 2003). Triterpenes in Eriobotrya Japonica have antifibrotic effects in pulmonary fibrosis (Yang et al., 2012).

	Huang Qin (Scutellaria Baicalensis)	Baicalein, chrysin, wogonin, and oroxylin A has therapeutic efficacy against acute lung injury caused by influenza A (H1N1) virus (Zhi et al., 2019).

Baicalin may bind to the ACE2 enzyme to block entry of SARS-CoV-2 (Chen & Du, 2020).

Chrysin may inhibit 3CL^{pro} and baicalin may inhibit PL^{pro} (Wu et al., 2020).

Scutellarin is predicted to bind to the ACE2 receptor to prevent SARS-CoV-2 entry (Chen & Du, 2020).

Scutellarein inhibits the helicase protein in SARS-CoV-1 (Yu et al., 2012).

Scutellarin suppresses NLP3 inflammasome activation in macrophages, decreases NFKB, IL-6, TNF-α, and IL-1β (Liu et al., 2018; Wang et al., 2016; Tan et al., 2016).

Scutellarin also protects against LPS induced aute lung injury via inhibition of NFKB activation in mice |

| | | (Tan et al., 2009). |

PHASE 4: RECOVERY STAGE FORMULA 1

1. SHENG MAI SAN – GENERATE THE PULSE POWDER

Upon recovering from a viral respiratory illness, if patients experience fatigue, low blood-oxygen saturation levels, and labored respiration after their fever is gone, it is time to consider *Sheng Mai San* to support Qi and Yin for Covid-19 (Chen, 2020). *Sheng Mai San* is a formula from *Nei Wai Shang Bian Huo Luo* (Clarification about Internal and External Disease Causation), published in 1247 by Li Dong Yuan (1180-1251 CE) (Dharmananda, 2001). *Sheng Mai San* (Generate the Pulse Powder) has traditionally been used for patients who suffered a severe illness, especially heart attack, congestive heart failure, or acute bronchitis, or blood pressure associated with cardiogenic or septic shock (ibid, 2001). *Sheng Mai San* can also be used to support the recovery of other respiratory illnesses, from the common cold to influenza, bronchitis, and pneumonia.

Sheng Mai San contains Ren Shen (Panax Ginseng), Mai Dong (Ophiopogon Japonicus), and Wu Wei Zi (Schisandra Chinensis). You may recall that the saponin, ginsenoside Rg1 derived from Ginseng, has been shown to improve LPS induced acute lung injury by inhibiting inflammatory responses and modulating infiltration of M2 macrophages (Bao et al., 2015). The ginsenoside Rg1 regulates innate immune responses in macrophages through differentially modulating NFKB and PI3K/Akt/mTOR pathways important for regulating the cell cycle (Wang et al., 2014). Also, Wu et al. (2020) found that ginsenoside-Rb1 inhibited SARS-CoV-1 replication at non-toxic concentrations.

Mai Dong (Ophiopogon Japonicus), commonly used for respiratory disorders, was found to be useful for respiratory symptoms in older adults (Cai et al., 2013). Also, schizandrin and deoxyschizandrin have been shown to inhibit mitogen-activated protein kinase (MAPK) and NFKB in acute airway viral infections (Eng et al., 2019). *Sheng Mai San* can be found in tablets and granule extracts or prepared as a decoction.

Sheng Mai San – Ingredients and Dosages
• Ren Shen (Radix Ginseng) 9g • Mai Dong (Ophiopogon Japonicus) 15g • Wu Wei Zi (Schisandra Chinensis) 9g

Preparation and dosage: It is best to soak herbs in 400 ml of water for 20 minutes before cooking. Bring the herbs up to a rolling boil and then lower to a simmer for 20-30 minutes. Each formula is to be taken warm in 2 divided doses between meals in the morning and evening.

The following chart describes the bioactive compounds and their actions in *Sheng Mai San*. Please note studies for each herb referenced in the chart below.

Sheng Mai San Ingredients, Bioactive Compounds, and Actions		
Herbs in Sheng Mai San	Herb Name	Bioactive Compounds and Actions
	Ren Shen (Radix Ginseng)	Ginsenoside Rg1 has been shown to improve LPS induced acute lung injury by inhibiting inflammatory responses and modulating infiltration of M2 macrophages (Bao et al., 2015). Ginsenoside Rg1 regulates innate immune responses in macrophages

		through differentially modulating NFKB, PI3K/Akt/mTOR signaling pathways important for regulating the cell cycle (Wang et al., 2014). Ginsenoside-Rb1 inhibited SARS-CoV-1 replication at non-toxic concentrations. (Wu et al., 2004).
	Mai Dong (Ophiopogon Japonicus)	Homoisoflavonoids (Lin et al., 2010). Effective for respiratory symptoms in older adults (Cai et al., 2013).
	Wu Wei Zi (Schisandra Chinensis)	Schizandrin Deoxyschizandrin Inhibits mitogen-activated protein kinase (MAPK) and NFKB in acute airway viral infections (Eng et al., 2019).

Phase 4: Recovery Stage Formula 2

2. SHA SHEN MAI DONG TANG - GLEHNIA AND OPHIOPOGONIS DECOCTION

Upon recovering from acute respiratory distress syndrome, especially in the case of Covid-19, patients may suffer from pulmonary fibrosis due to lung tissue damage caused by the viral infection and the immune system's response

(Spagnolo et al., 2020). In this case, *Sha Shen Mai Dong Tang,* or a modified version of this formula, may be considered depending on the presentation. The traditional formula, *Sha Shen Mai Dong Tang,* also comes from Wu Tang's Qing Dynasty 1798 text, *Wen Bing Tiao Bian* (Systematic Differentiation of Warm Diseases).

If Qi (energy) and Yin (fluids) depletion exist along with Lung and Spleen (digestion) deficiency symptoms of thirst and poor digestion, the following formula may be helpful.

Sha Shen Mai Dong Tang – Ingredients and Dosages	
• Sha Shen (Radix Glehniae) 15g • Mai Dong (Radix Ophiopogonis) 15g • Yu Zhu (Aromatic Solomon's Seal Rhizome) 15g • Sang Ye (Folium Mori) 12g	• Bai Bian Dou (Semen Lablab Album) 10g • Tian Hua Fen, (Radix Trichosanthis) 15g • Gan Cao (Radix Glycyrrhizae) 10g

If there is scarring of the lung tissue, lung function may also be compromised, which can lead to symptoms of wheezing and dyspnea. In this case, patients may still require ventilator support in the hospital. If patients still feel weak upon returning from the hospital, they may benefit from herbs that help build Qi and Yin (energy and fluids) and restore the Spleen and Lung function (Chen, 2020). In this case, practitioners can consider a modified *Sha Shen Mai Dong Tang* (Glehnia and Ophiopogonis Decoction). This modified version, suggested by Dr. John Chen, includes the *Sheng Mai San* prescription described above to increase the Qi (energy) and Yin (fluids) nourishing effects.

Modified Sha Shen Mai Dong Tang + Sheng Mai San Ingredients and Dosages	
• Sha Shen (Radix Glehniae) 15g • Mai Dong (Radix Ophiopogonis) 15g • Wu Wei Zi (Fructus Schisandrae Chinensis) 15g	• Zi Su Zi (Fructus Perillae) 12g • Zhe Bei Mu (Bulbus Fritillariae Thunbergii) 12g • Ku Xing Ren (Semen Armeniacae

• Ren Shen (Radix et Rhizoma Ginseng) 12g • Lai Fu Zi (Semen Raphani) 15g • Si Gua Luo (Retinervus Luffae Fructus) 15g • Ju Luo (Vascular Citri Reticulatae) 15g	Amarum) 12g • Huang Qin (Radix Scutellariae) 15g • Gan Cao (Radix Glycyrrhizae) 10g

Preparation and dosage: It is best to soak herbs in 400 ml of water for 20 minutes before cooking. Bring the herbs up to a rolling boil and then lower to a simmer for 20-30 minutes. Each formula is to be taken warm in 2 divided doses between meals in the morning and evening.

SAFETY OF MEDICINAL HERBS

Now that we have explored the potential benefits of Chinese herbs for viral respiratory infections, we need to consider the safety of medicinal herbs. Herbs are generally recognized as safe, but practitioners need to heed caution in treating viral respiratory illnesses et al. disorders. For example, the herb Kuan Dong Hua (Flos Farfarae) is included in the formula *Qing Fei Pai Du Tang*. But since it has been reported that this herb contains pyrrolizidine alkaloids (senkirkine and senecionine), which are potentially hepatotoxic and carcinogenic, astute practitioners would want to avoid using this herb in general and especially for patients who have liver problems. Zi Wan (Radix et Rhizoma Asteris) can also be hepatotoxic with extended use and should only be used for short periods in general and not at all for patients who have liver problems (Peng et al., 2016). Dryopteris Crassirhizoma (Guan Zhong) is also considered to be slightly toxic and also needs to be used with caution (Dharmananda, 2003).

Also, some compounds such as baicalin in Huang Qin (Scutellaria Baicalensis) may magnify or oppose the effect of pharmaceuticals and should be carefully evaluated for those on medications (Tian et al., 2013; Fong et al., 2015). As mentioned previously, practitioners should also heed caution in using herbs like Huang Qi (Astragalus Membranaceus), Echinacea (Echinacea Purpurea), Ren

Shen (Radix Ginseng), and Chuan Xin Lian (Andrographis Paniculata) in patients with autoimmune disease. Practitioners are also encouraged to thoroughly check for hidden allergens in the formulas they are recommending for those with food allergies or sensitivities to ingredients such as soy (Dan Dou Chi) and tree nuts such as Ku Xing Ren (Semen Armeniacae Amarum).

PART III

The Role of Phytochemistry and Nutrition

Given the research that we have explored, practitioners can now consider the role of herbal and dietary flavonoids as functional foods for respiratory infections. Functional foods refer to foods that enhance specific physiological responses to promote health. The profound antiviral, immune-modulating and anti-inflammatory effects of enhanced phytonutrition with dietary flavonoids may help bring tremendous relief to those struggling with immune dysregulation and inflammation caused by viral respiratory illnesses.

Combining potent plant compounds (including flavonoids from foods and medicinal herbs) helps supply the key ingredients to the immune system that may block viral entry, inhibit viral replication, and modulate immune/inflammatory responses. The more we understand each plant's actions and synergistic use of these compounds (in herbs and foods), the more we can personalize combinations to shore up our patient's defenses and improve their health.

NUTRIGENOMICS - MODULATING NFKB AND CYTOKINES

Nutrigenomics is the science that studies the role of nutrition on gene expression. In this book, we have been considering the role of potent plant compounds such as flavonoids, kaempferol, quercetin, and luteolin as antiviral, immune-modulating, and anti-inflammatory agents. These herbal compounds, which are also in common fruits and vegetables, act on a critical gene transcription factor called Nuclear Factor Kappa B (NFKB).

NFKB is a protein that acts as a switch to turn inflammation either "on" or "off" when cells sense "danger" in the form of infections, emotional, and metabolic stress. Activation of NFKB is required for transcription of the genes for many of the proinflammatory mediators associated with acute respiratory distress syndrome (Horowitz et al., 2020). If this protein group is overactive, it will continually produce the inflammation response where none is needed. In Covid-19 patients, activation of NFKB (and the NLRP3 inflammasome) yields an unbridled production of proinflammatory cytokines, such as IL-6, TNF-α, and IL-1β.

Understanding how to counteract this expression with herbs and foods, once these switches get turned "on," may help decrease inflammation and the cytokine storm. Getting rid of infections by inhibiting viral attachment and replication is the first step in preventing NFKB from turning on the inflammatory cascade. Yet, once inflammation is excessive in Covid-19 and other viral respiratory infections, it makes sense to include natural agents that modulate NFKB and cytokine overexpression. The critical point is that we need to apply the most advanced strategies to tame hyperimmune responses and resultant inflammation effectively.

As we have seen, polyphenols and other plant compounds in medicinal herbs have the power to bind to and turn "off" nuclear transcription factors (which turn "off" inflammatory genes). A combination of polyphenols from foods and medicinal herbs may also help block viral entry, inhibit viral replication, and regulate the immune/inflammatory processes. Given this information, we can encourage the inclusion of flavonoids from fruits, vegetables, and teas that can epigenetically change gene transcription via inhibiting NFKB and cytokine production. Besides herbal medicine, this includes dietary flavonoids and other natural compounds that target anti-inflammatory gene transcription factors like NFKB. In effect, these potent compounds exert their epigenetic impact through NFKB inhibition, improved DNA methylation, and histone modification, resulting in less inflammation and overall symptom improvement.

COMMON NFKB INHIBITORS

We now know that effective NFKB inhibitors are available from foods, herbal medicine, and essential oils. The following NFKB inhibitors are promising candidates for chronic inflammation.

Common NFKB Inhibitors	
• Allicin in garlic and ginger	• Sulforaphane (found in cruciferous vegetables)
• Curcumin in turmeric	• Vitamins A, C, D, E
• ECGC and theanine in green tea	• Berberine in Scutellaria Baicalensis
• Ginkgolides in gingko biloba	• Kaempferol in kale, chives
• Melatonin in mushrooms	• Luteolin in celery, thyme
• Quercetin in dill, oregano, onions, leeks, citrus, spinach	• Lipoic acid in spinach, broccoli, yams
• Resveratrol in grapes, red wine	• Zinc in oysters
• Silymarin in milk thistle	• EPA/DHA in fish and algae
• Carnosol in rosemary	• Gingerols in ginger
• Selenium in Brazil nuts	• Myrcene in lavender and frankincense essential oil
• Limonene in lemon, orange, and grapefruit essential oils	• Alpha-pinene in pine, sage, and eucalyptus essential oils

THE GUT-LUNG AXIS AND PHYTONUTRIENT DENSE FOODS

Interestingly, recent research suggests a critical role for the crosstalk between gut microbiota and the lungs, known as gut–lung axis (Zhang et al., 2020). Extensive studies have observed alterations in the gut microbial species and metabolites in lung diseases, including pneumonia, allergy, asthma, and lung cancer (Zhang et al., 2020). We also know that flavonoid intake on the gut microbial community structure affects intestinal and systemic inflammation and the metabolic response (Cassidy and Minehane, 2017). Since changes in the gut microbiome have been linked to changes in immune-inflammation responses and disease development in the lungs, it is possible that including flavonoids in the diet is a potential strategy to manipulate the gut microbiota as the therapeutic approach for lung diseases (Zhang et al., 2020).

Many common flavonoids can be found in our diet. For example, many antiviral, anti-inflammatory, and immune-modulating compounds found in Chinese herbs, including luteolin, quercetin, luteolin, naringenin, apigenin, oleuropein, curcumin, catechin, and epicatechin-gallate, can also be sourced from foods. In studying the foods that contain these compounds, astute practitioners can consider foods in the same manner as they recommend herbal medicines. The most important ones for a synergistic effect might include the same active compounds in the herbs practitioners use for viral respiratory infections. For example, the following herbs and foods are rich in an array of flavonoids with antiviral effects (Khaerunnisa et al., 2020).

Herbs and Foods Rich in Flavonoids	
• Kaempferol –Ma Huang • Quercetin– Xiang Chun Ye • Luteolin—Zi Hua Di Ding • Naringenin - Zhi Shi • Apigenin—Bo He • Oleuropein –Qing Guo • Curcumin - Yu Jin, Jiang Huang, E Zhu • Catechin and ECGC - Lu Cha	• Kaempferol -Leeks • Quercetin-Onions • Luteolin-Celery • Naringenin-Citrus • Apigenin-Mint, parsley • Oleuropein-Olives, olive oil and olive leaves • Curcumin • Green Tea
(Source: Khaerunnisa et al., 2020)	

The growing evidence of the beneficial effects of dietary flavonoids on health is undeniable. Now let's hone in on food sources of the top three antiviral flavonoids, i.e., kaempferol, quercetin, and luteolin found in medicinal herbs and foods. Pay attention to the foods and herbs that contain more than one of these flavonoids.

Flavonols: Kaempferol

A member of the flavonols, kaempferol, is found in many medicinal herbs and common foods such as spinach, kale, broccoli, dill, chives, and green tea. Besides antiviral activity, kaempferol in brassica vegetables is well known for inhibiting cancer, reducing heart disease risk, and has proven antimicrobial and anti-allergic properties (Schwarz et al., 2014; Calderón-Montaño et al., 2011). Kaempferol and quercetin both exhibit anti-inflammatory actions through the inhibition of the phospholipase A2 (via arachidonic acid), lipoxygenase, cyclooxygenase, and thromboxane enzymes, and the modulation of iNOS thereby inhibiting NO production (Santangelo et al., 2007; Yoon & Baek, 2005).

Kaempferol was also shown to regulate MAPK and NFKB signaling pathways to attenuate LPS-induced acute lung injury in mice (Chen et al., 2012).

Kaempferol also acts on targets such as TNF-α to modulate systemic inflammation and oxidative stress (Yang et al., 2015). Khaerunnisa et al. (2020) found that quercetin, along with kaempferol and luteolin, was predicted to inhibit the main protease (M^{pro}) in SARS-CoV-2.

All of these effects make kaempferol a stellar candidate for viral respiratory infections. However, without further studies, we can't assume that kaempferol (or luteolin, or quercetin) from foods alone will block SARS-CoV-2. However, combining kaempferol and other phytonutrient dense foods hold out the possibility of being very useful. The following charts note the many herbs and foods that contain kaempferol.

Herbs That Contain Kaempferol	
• Sang Ye (Folium Mori) • Mian Ma Guan Zhong (Dryopteris Crassirhizoma) • Ma Huang (Herba Ephedrae) • Bo He (Herba Menthae) • Huang Qi (Astragalus membranaceus) • Lian Qiao (Fructus Forsythiae) • Pi Pa Ye (Eriobotryae Folium)	• Lian Qiao (Fructus Forsythiae) • Jin Yin Hua (Flos Lonicerae Japonicae) • Ju Hua (Flos Chrysanthemi) • Hong Jing Tian (Radix et Rhizoma Rhodiola Crenulata)

Foods That Contain Kaempferol

To synergize the potent effect of herbs, we can also recommend foods rich in kaempferol.

Foods That Contain Kaempferol	
• Capers • Spinach • Kale • Dill • Chives • Tarragon • Saffron • Fennel leaves • Broccoli • Asparagus • Strawberries • Blueberries • Gooseberries • Watermelon • Kiwi • Apricot	• Blackberries • Bananas • Peach • Cherries • Apples • Watercress • Mustard greens • Arugula • Endive • Cabbage • Turnip greens • Soybeans • Chia seeds • Nuts • Beans • Green Tea
(Sources: Bhagwat et al., 2011 U.S. Department of Agriculture; Dabeek & Marra 2019; Miean & Mohammad, 2001).	

Quercetin

Another flavonol, quercetin, is found in numerous medicinal Chinese herbs and as well as in many common foods. Perhaps, increasing the amount of quercetin in foods may be as important as the herbs we use for their antiviral and immune-modulating effects. Quercetin affects immunity and inflammation by acting mainly on leukocytes and targeting intracellular signaling kinases, enzymes, and membrane proteins crucial for cellular specific functions (Chirimbolo, 2010). Quercetin also has a protective effect on cells and has been shown to successfully attenuate oxidative epithelial cell injury in lung inflammation (Hayashi et al., 2012). Khaerunnisa et al. (2020) also found that quercetin, along with kaempferol and luteolin, was predicted to inhibit the main protease (M^{pro}) in SARS-CoV-2.

Without further studies, we can't assume that quercetin (or kaempferol or luteolin) from foods alone will block SARS-CoV-2. However, combining quercetin-based herbs et al. functional flavonoids hold out the possibility of being very useful. The following herbs and functional foods that contain quercetin can be considered for their antiviral, anti-inflammatory, and immune-modulating effects in Covid-19 and other viral respiratory illnesses.

Herbs That Contain Quercetin

Herbs That Contain Quercetin	
<ul><li>Xiang Chun Ye (Toona Sinensis Roem)</li><li>Ma Huang (Herba Ephedrae)</li><li>Zi Hua Di Ding (Herba Violae)</li><li>Bo He (Herba Menthae)</li><li>Hu Zhang (Rhizoma Polygoni Cuspidati)</li><li>Jin Yin Hua (Flos Lonicerae Japonicae)</li><li>Lian Qiao (Fructus Forsythiae)</li><li>Pi Pa Ye (Eriobotryae Folium)</li><li>Da Zao (Zizyphus Jujubae)</li></ul>	<ul><li>Yu Xing Cao (Houttuynia Cordata)</li><li>Ju Hua (Flos Chrysanthemi)</li><li>Sang Ye (Folium Mori)</li><li>Zi Wan (Radix et Rhizoma Asteris)</li><li>Hong Jing Tian (Radix et Rhizoma Rhodiola Crenulata)</li></ul>

Foods That Contain Quercetin

To synergize the potent effect of herbs, we can also recommend foods rich in quercetin.

Foods That Contain Quercetin	
<ul><li>Dill</li><li>Mexican oregano</li><li>Chili peppers</li><li>Yellow onions, cooked</li></ul>	<ul><li>Mustard greens</li><li>Cranberry</li><li>Collard greens</li><li>Scallions</li></ul>

• Red onions, raw • Spring onions • Spinach • Kale • Fennel leaves • Red leaf lettuce • Broccoli • Watercress • Cilantro • Arugula • Asparagus • Leeks • Radicchio	• Cherry • Blueberry • Blackberry • Figs • Apples • Grapes • Citrus • Capers • Red wine • Elderberries • Litchi fruit • Green Tea • Black tea
(Sources: Bhagwat et al., 2011 U.S. Department of Agriculture; Dabeek & Marra 2019; Miean & Mohammad, 2001).	

Flavones: Luteolin

Luteolin is a flavone in many herbs in the TCM pharmacy that have antiviral, immune modulating, and anti-inflammatory effects. Luteolin is an excellent candidate for viral respiratory illnesses and has been shown to attenuate the inflammatory response to endotoxin-induced acute lung injury (ALI) in mice via inhibition of MAPK and NFKB pathways and antioxidant effects (Kuo et al., 2011). Considering the overexpression of cytokines seen in viral respiratory infections, and the fact that luteolin suppresses NFKB production of the inflammatory cytokines TNF-α and IL-6 (Kang et al., 2010), we might consider including more luteolin in the diet to modulate this response.

Like quercetin and kaempferol, luteolin also causes inhibition of iNOS and NO production (Santangelo et al., 2007). Luteolin and quercetin have been shown to decrease pro-inflammatory cytokines such as TNF-α and IL-1, and modulate lymphocytes and neutrophils (Kim et al., 2004; Coutinho et al., 2009). Khaerunnisa et al. (2020) found that luteolin, along with quercetin, and kaempferol, were predicted to inhibit the main protease (M^{pro}) in SARS-CoV-

2.

Without further studies, we can't assume that luteolin or kaempferol, or quercetin from foods alone will also block M^{pro} in SARS-CoV-2. However, adding foods that contain these flavonoids hold out the possibility of being very useful. The following herbs and functional foods that contain luteolin can be considered for their antiviral, anti-inflammatory, and immune-modulating effects in Covid-19 and other viral respiratory illnesses.

Herbs That Contain Luteolin

Herbs That Contain Luteolin	
• Ju Hua (Flos Chrysanthemi) • Xiang Ru (Herba Moslae) • Ma Huang (Herba Ephedrae) • Zi Hua Di Ding (Herba Violae) • Hong Jing Tian (Radix et Rhizoma Rhodiola Crenulata)	• Lian Qiao (Fructus Forsythiae) • Jin Yin Hua (Flos Lonicerae Japonicae) • Yu Xing Cao (Houttuynia Cordata)

Foods That Contain Luteolin

To synergize the potent effect of herbs, we can also recommend foods rich in quercetin.

Foods That Contain Luteolin	
• Olives • Radicchio • Chicory greens • Pumpkin • Red leaf lettuce • Artichoke • Kohlrabi • Broccoli	• Celery • Green peppers • Thyme • Chamomile • Dandelion • Spring onions • Leeks • Parsley

> (Sources: Bhagwat et al., 2011 U.S. Department of Agriculture; Miean & Mohammad, 2001).

GLUTATHIONE, N-ACETYL-CYSTEINE, AND ALPHA-LIPOIC ACID

Glutathione (GSH), N-acetyl-cysteine (NAC), and alpha-lipoic acid (ALA) have all been shown to regulate NFKB signaling (Suzuki et al., 1992; Kachigian et al., 1997). GSH is the most important antioxidant that is present in every cell of the body. Glutathione depletion is common in viral infections with inflammation in the lungs (Ghezzi, 2011). In one recent study, oral and IV glutathione, glutathione precursors (N-acetyl-cysteine), and alpha-lipoic acid all helped to inhibit NFKB and decrease respiratory distress in two Covid-19 patients with dyspnea and pneumonia (Horowitz et al., 2020).

A controlled clinical trial of NAC demonstrated that patients with ARDS had depressed plasma and red cell glutathione concentrations, which increased substantially after intravenous NAC (Bernard et al., 1990). Clinical responses included increased oxygen delivery, improved lung compliance, and pulmonary edema (ibid, 1990).

While intravenous NAC, glutathione, and alpha-lipoic acid therapy can be explored with a qualified doctor, many plant-based precursors to glutathione may also be useful. Plant-based compounds that act as building blocks of glutathione include cysteine from sulfur-rich allium and cruciferous vegetables, which may raise and maintain their level inside and outside of cells. Alpha-lipoic acid is also one of the most well known naturally occurring compounds for enhancing intracellular glutathione for potent antiviral, antioxidant, and anti-inflammatory effects (Baur et al., 1991; Tibullo et al., 2017).

Plant Sources to Increase Glutathione	
• Garlic • Onion • Broccoli • Kale • Collards • Cabbage • Brussels sprouts	• Leeks • Chives • Mustard greens • Avocado • Cauliflower • Sweet potatoes • Watercress
(Bruce & Grossan 2007; Gottfried, 2019)	

Plant Sources of Alpha-Lipoic Acid	
• Spinach • Broccoli • Yams • Potatoes	• Tomatoes • Brussels sprouts • Carrots • Beets
(Mijnhout, 2010)	

MANNOSE-BINDING LECTINS

Practitioners can also consider food sources of mannose-binding lectins to maximize antiviral, and immune-modulating effects. Mannose-binding lectins (MBL) are important molecules created by the innate immune system that function as an ante-antibody before the specific antibody response (Ip et al., 2005). In this regard, food sources of mannose-binding lectins may help improve innate immunity.

Mannose-binding lectins have been shown to penetrate and break down the coronaviruses glycoprotein shells (Keyaerts et al., 2007). Keyaerts et al. (2007) also demonstrated MBL's target viral attachment and revealed food sources of mannose-binding lectins that effectively penetrate and break down the glycoprotein shells of SARS-CoV-1, including leeks and nettles. Interestingly, Ip et al. (2005) demonstrated a higher number of MBL gene polymorphisms in patients with SARS-CoV-1 with a higher frequency of haplotypes associated with low serum levels of mannose-binding lectins in patients with SARS-CoV-1 than in control subjects. They also found serum levels of MBL's to be significantly lower in patients with SARS-CoV-1 than in control subjects (Ip et al., 2005). Without further studies on mannose-binding lectins for SARS-CoV-2, at this point, we can't yet say that MBL's are inhibitors of SARS-CoV-2. In any case, nettles and leeks are very nutritious and make a great addition to any healthy diet.

Supplements

While an anti-inflammatory diet is usually sufficient, immune-compromised patients may want to top off their reserves with a few supplements that have known antiviral and immune-modulating effects, e.g., vitamin C, D, Zinc, probiotics, and melatonin. To broadly cover immunocompetency, practitioners can also recommend B vitamins, especially B2, B6, B12, and folate.

FINAL THOUGHTS

Integrative treatments are urgently needed to manage Severe Acute Respiratory Syndrome (SARS)-CoV-2 in the United States and elsewhere. Practitioners, such as acupuncturists trained in herbal medicine, and other concerned providers, including naturopaths, doctors, and functional medicine specialists, may all be able to offer profound supportive therapy for non-hospitalized patients suffering from viral respiratory illnesses, such as the dreaded seasonal flu, asthma, bronchitis, pneumonia, and Covid-19.

To offer the best possible care to patients, all integrative medicine practitioners can learn more about the antiviral, immune-modulating, and anti-inflammatory effects of medicinal herbs used to treat viral respiratory illnesses. Until we have randomized controlled trials to demonstrate the efficacy of medicinal herbs for Covid-19, we can consider the current empirical results for this safe and supportive therapy in this and other epidemics.

Hopefully, the anti-SARS-CoV-2 activity of traditional herbal compounds will be published shortly, and a viable remedy will receive scientific validation. Until then, we can study the research about the potent compounds in herbs used for SARS-CoV-1 and other viral respiratory infections, as well as current network pharmacology analyses of herbs and formulas, plus molecular docking and virtual screening studies for SARS-CoV-2. We can also consider using empirically proven herbal remedies and phytonutrient dense foods to support patients suffering from Covid-19 and other viral respiratory illnesses.

About Anne Angelone, MSTCM, DACM, Licensed Acupuncturist

I spent the first seven years of my career treating thousands of patients at community clinics during the AIDS crisis here in San Francisco, CA. During that time, and throughout my career of specializing in autoimmune disease, I took a lot of classes and gained a lot of experience, knowledge, and insight about nutrition and immune modulation. I have written books about dietary interventions for autoimmune disease, and I recently developed a scalp acupuncture model for autoimmune, neuropsychological, neurobehavioral, and neurodegenerative diseases.

Like every other acupuncturist on the planet, I have reviewed the current herbal medicine recommendations for Covid-19. I was surprised by the amount of research on the role of flavonoids and other plant compounds for viral respiratory illnesses. The idea for this book stemmed from the need to clarify the role of potent plant compounds for viral respiratory infections in general and to investigate what compounds might be similarly useful for SARS-CoV-2 in particular. Besides acupuncturists and TCM herbalists, this book is for all practitioners who want to learn more about the potent compounds found in traditional herbal formulas used for viral respiratory infections.

Ultimately, in my opinion, medicinal herbs and functional foods may prove to be a sound supportive therapy for Covid-19 patients, especially when hospitalization is deemed unnecessary. With more research, herbal formulas that help speed recovery in patients who still suffer from respiratory distress, fatigue, and poor digestion upon recovering from Covid-19 will also likely be scientifically validated. I hope that, given the concise information in this book, integrative practitioners around the globe may be able to help decrease the severity of symptoms associated viral respiratory infections that do not require hospitalization.

I am very grateful for the leadership, guidance, and extensive translations by John Chen Ph.D., OMD, L.Ac., in his lectures and from Dr. Chen and Lori Hsu, MTOM, MS., in their excellent work, "How Covid-19 (2019-nCoV) is Currently Treated in China with TCM" (2020). It is also inspiring to learn from the countless practitioners who are considering the most effective strategies for Covid-19. I also want to thank my colleagues, Annette Kohl, DACM, L.Ac., and Liat Barnea, MS., L.Ac. for their help and encouragement in writing this book.

Finally, thank you for taking the time to read Functional Herbal Medicine and Phytonutrition. We can and are doing this together. For more information about my other books and continuing education classes that I have created for CA Licensed Acupuncturists, please visit my website at anneangelone.com.

References

Abourashed, E.A., El-Alfy, A.T., Khan, I.A., & Walker, L. (2003). Ephedra in perspective—A current review. *Phytotherapy Research*, 17, 703–712.

Ahmed, H.M. (2019, January). Ethnomedicinal, Phytochemical and Pharmacological Investigations of Perilla frutescens (L.) Britt. *Molecules*, 24(1):102.doi: 10.3390/molecules24010102

Alves, D.S., Perez-Fons, L., & Estepa, A. (2004). Membrane-related effects underlying the biological activity of the anthraquinones emodin and barbaloin, *Biochemical Pharmacology*, 68:549-561.

Ahn, K.S., Noh, E.J., Cha, K.H., Kim, Y.S., Lim, S.S., Shin, K.H., & Jung, S.H. (2006). Inhibitory effects of Irigenin from the rhizomes of Belamcandae chinensis on nitric oxide and prostaglandin E(2) production in murine macrophage RAW 264.7 cells. *Life Sciences*, 78, 2336–2342.

Asif, M. (2011, March). Health effects of omega-3,6,9 fatty acids: Perilla frutescens is a good example of plant oils. *Oriental Pharmacy and Experimental Medicine*, 11(1):51-59.

Avendaño, C., & Menéndez, J.C. in *Medicinal Chemistry of Anticancer Drugs* (Second Edition), 2015.

Aziz, N., Kim, M.Y., & Cho, J.Y. (2018, May). Anti-inflammatory effects of luteolin: A review of in vitro, in vivo, and in silico studies. *Journal of Ethnopharmacology*, vol 225, pp. 342-358. DOI:10.1016/j.jeep.2018.05.019

Azam, S., Jakaria, M., Kim, I.S., Kim, J., Haque, M., & Choi, D.K. (2019). Regulation of Toll-Like Receptor (TLR) Signaling Pathway by Polyphenols: Focus on TLR4 Signaling. *Frontiers in Immunology*, 10. 10.3389/fimmu.2019.01000.

Bai, Y., Zheng, Y.J., Pang, W.J., Peng, W., Wu, H., Yao, H.L.,…Su, W.W. (2018). Identification and Comparison of Constituents of Aurantii Fructus and Aurantii Fructus Immaturus by UFLC-DAD-Triple TOF-MS/MS. *Molecules*, 23(4), 803. MDPI AG. http://dx.doi.org/10.3390/molecules23040803

Ballantyne, S. (2017). *Paleo Principles*. Victory Belt Publishing.

Bao, S., Zou, Y., Wang, B., Li, Y., Zhu, J., Luo, Y., & Li, J. (2015). Ginsenoside Rg1 improves lipopolysaccharide-induced acute lung injury by inhibiting inflammatory responses and modulating infiltration of M2 macrophages. *International Immunopharmacology*, 28 (1), pp. 429-434.

Baur, A., Harrer, T., Peukert, M., Jahn, G., Kalden, J.R., & Fleckenstein, B. (1991). Alpha-lipoic acid is an effective inhibitor of human immuno-deficiency virus (HIV-1) replication. *Wiener Klinische Wochenschrift, 69*:722-724. https://doi.org/10.1007/bf01649442

Bensky, D. & Barolet, R. *Formulas and Strategies*, Eastland Press, 1990.

Bernard, G.R. (1990). Potential of N-acetylcysteine as treatment for the adult respiratory distress syndrome. *European Respiratory Journal*, 11:496s–498s.

Bhagwat, S., Haytowitz, D.B., & Holden, J.M. (2011, September). Nutrient Data Laboratory Beltsville Human Nutrition Research Center Agricultural Research Service. U.S. Department of Agriculture.

Boustie, J., Stigliani, J.L., Montanha, J., Amoros, M., Payard, M., & Girre, L. (1998 April) Antipoliovirus structure-activity relationships of some aporphine alkaloids. *Journal of Natural Products*, 61(4):480-4

Brahmkshatriya, P.P. & Brahmkshatriya, P.S. (2013, May). Terpenes: Chemistry, Biological Role, and Therapeutic Applications. *Natural Products*. pp. 2665-2691.

Bratkov, V.M., Shkondrov, A.M., Zdraveva, P.K., & Krasteva, I.N. (2016). Flavonoids from the genus Astragalus: Phytochemistry and biological activity. *Pharmacognosy Reviews*, 10:11-32.

Bruce, D.F., & Grossan, M. (2007). *The Sinus Cure*. Ballantine Books.

Cai, Y., Shi, R., Song, H.J., Shang, M.L., Shen, T., Shariff, M.,…Rao, J.Y. (2013, May). Effects of Lung Support Formula on respiratory symptoms among older adults: results of a three-month follow-up study in Shanghai, China. *Nutrition Journal*, 12: 57. DOI: 10.1186/1475-2891-12-57

Calderón-Montaño, J.M., Burgos-Morón, E., Pérez-Guerrero, C., & López-Lázaro, M. (2011, April). A review on the dietary flavonoid kaempferol. *Mini Reviews in Medical Chemistry*, (4):298-344.

Cassidy, A., & Minihane, A. M. (2017). The role of metabolism (and the microbiome) in defining the clinical efficacy of dietary flavonoids. *The American Journal of Clinical Nutrition*, 105(1), 10–22. https://doi.org/10.3945/ajcn.116.136051

Chadwick, M., Trewin, H., Gawthrop, F., & Wagstaff, C. (2013, June). Sesquiterpenoids Lactones: Benefits to Plants and People. *International Journal of Molecular Sciences*, 14(6): 12780–12805. DOI: 10.3390/ijms140612780

Chang, H.Y., Chen, Y.C., Lin, J.G., Lin, I.H., Huang, H.F., Yeh, C.C.,…Huang, G.J. (2018). Asatone prevents acute lung injury by reducing expressions of NFKB, MAPK and inflammatory cytokines. *American Journal of Chinese Medicine*, 46 (3), pp. 651-671

Chan, K.W., Wang, V.T., & Tang, S.C.W. (2020, March). Covid-19: An Update on the Epidemiological, Clinical, Preventive and Therapeutic Evidence and Guidelines of Integrative Chinese–Western Medicine for the Management of 2019 Novel Coronavirus Disease. *The American Journal of Chinese Medicine*, Vol. 48, No. 3, 1–26.

Chao, L.K., Hua, K.F., Hsu, H.Y., Cheng, S.S., Lin, L.F., Chen, C.J., & Chen, S.T. (2008). Cinnamaldehyde inhibits proinflammatory cytokines secretion from monocytes/macrophages through suppression of intracellular signaling. *Food and Chemical Toxicology*, 46, 220–231.

Chao, W.W., and Lin, B.F. (2010, May). Isolation and identification of bioactive compounds in Andrographis paniculata (Chuan Xin Lian). *Chinese Medicine,* 2010; 5: 17 May 13. DOI: 10.1186/1749-8546-5-17

Chen, C.J., Michaelis, M., Hsu, H.K., Tsai, C.C., Yang, K., Wu, Y.C., Cinatl, J., & Doerr, H.W. (2008). Toona Sinensis Roem tender leaf extract inhibits SARS-Coronavirus replication. *Journal of Ethnopharmacology*, 120.108-11. 10.1016/j.jep.2008.07.048

Chen, H., & Du, Q. (2020). Potential Natural Compounds for Preventing

2019-nCoV Infection. *Preprints.org.* 2020010358.

Chen, I.Y., Moriyama, M., Chang, M.F. & Ichinohe, T. (2019). Severe Acute Respiratory Syndrome Coronavirus Viroporin 3a Activates the NLRP3 Inflammasome. *Frontiers in Microbiology*, 10:50. DOI: 10.3389/fmicb.2019.00050

Chen J. *In China: TCM (Traditional Chinese Medicine) for COVID19 with Dr. John Chen.* [Audio file]. With Dr. Kara Fitzgerald and Dr. John Chen. https://www.drkarafitzgerald.com/2020/04/01/episode-80-in-china-tcm-traditional-chinese-medicine-for-covid19-with-dr-john-chen/

Chen, J. [Lotus Institute aka elotus] (Mar 17, 2020). *How Coronavirus (COVID-19) is treated with TCM in China by Dr. John Chen, PharmD, PhD, OMD, L.Ac.* [Video file]. https://www.youtube.com/watch?v=BGcsFzKLdTI

Chen, J., & Hsu, L. (2020). How Covid-19 (2019-nCoV) is Currently Treated in China with TCM. Compiled, Translated and Edited by John K. Chen, Pharm.D., PhD., OMD, LAc. and Lori Hsu, MTOM, MS. TCM Resources for Coping with Covid-19 published on eLotus.org

Chen, J.J., Huang, C.C., Chang, H.Y., Li, P.Y., Liang, Y.C., Deng, J.S.,…Huang, G.J. (2017). Scutellaria baicalensis ameliorates acute lung injury by suppressing inflammation in vitro and in vivo. *American Journal of Chinese Medicine*, 45 (01), pp. 137-157.

Chen, L., Fan, J., Li, Y., Shi, X., Ju, D., Yan, Q.,…Zhu, H. (2014). Modified Jiu Wei Qiang Huo decoction improves dysfunctional metabolomics in influenza A pneumonia-infected mice. *Biomedical Chromatography*, 28(4), 468–474.

Chen, X.J., Yang, X.F., Liu, T.J., Guan, M.F., Feng, X.R, Dong, W.,…Sun, J.L. (2012). Kaempferol regulates MAPKs and NF-kappaB signaling pathways to attenuate LPS-induced acute lung injury in mice. *International Immunopharmacology*, 14, 209–216.

Chen, Y.J., Dong, J.J., Liu, J., Xu, W.X., Wei, Z.Y., Li, Y.T.,…Xiao, H. (2019). Network Pharmacology-Based Investigation of Protective Mechanism of Aster tataricus on Lipopolysaccharide-Induced Acute Lung Injury. International journal of molecular sciences, 20(3), 543.

Chen, Y., Liu, Q., Guo, D.J. (2020). Emerging coronaviruses: genome structure, replication, and pathogenesis. *Journal of Medical Virology*, 92:418–423.

Chen, Z., Du, X., Yang, Y., Cui, X., Zhang, Z., & Li, Y. (2018). Comparative study of chemical composition and active components against α-glucosidase of various medicinal parts of Morus alba L. *Biomedical Chromatography: BMC*, 32(11), e4328. https://doi.org/10.1002/bmc.4328

Cheng, P.W. Ng, L.T., Chiang, L.C., & Lin, C.C. (2006). Antiviral effects of saikosaponins on human coronavirus 229E in vitro. *Clinical and experimental pharmacology & physiology*, 33. 612-6. 10.1111/j.1440-1681.2006.04415.x.

Cheng, Y., Mai, J.Y., Hou, T.L., Ping, J., & Chen, J.J. (2016, February). Antiviral activities of atractylon from Atractylodis Rhizoma. *Journal of Integrative Medicine*, pp: 3704-3710. https://doi.org/10.3892/mmr.2016.5713

Chia, Y.H. Components of Toona Sinensis: review. In: Hsu H.K., Wong C.F., editors. Taiwan Toona. The R&D Country Club of Toona Sinensis; Kaohsiung, Taiwan: 2007. pp. 130–138.

Chin, Y.W., Jung, Y.H., Chae, H.S., Yoon, K.D., & Kim, J.W. (2011). Anti-inflammatory Constituents from the Roots of Saposhnikovia divaricata. Bulletin of Korean Chemistry Society, Vol. 32, No. 6 Notes DOI 10.5012/bkcs.2011.32.6.2132

Chiow, K.H., Phoon, M.C., Putti, T., Tan, B.K., Chow, V.T. (2016). Evaluation of activities of Houttuynia Cordata Thunb. Extract, quercetin, quercetrin and cinanserin on murine coronavirus and dengue virus infection. *Asian Pacific Journal of Tropical Medicine*, 9(1):1–7.

Chirumbolo, S. (2010, September). The role of quercetin, flavonols and flavones in modulating inflammatory cell function. *Inflammation and Allergy Drug Targets*, 9(4):263-85.

Choi, S.E., Yoon, J.H., Park, K.H., Kim, K.Y., Song, Y.J., Jin, H.Y., & Lee, M.W. (2014). Whitening activity of phenolic compounds from rhizome of Phragmites communis. *Natural Product Sciences*, 20. 269-273.

Cinatl, J., Morgenstern, B., Bauer, G., Chandra, P., Rabenau, H., & Doerr, H.W. (2003). Glycyrrhizin, an active component of liquorice roots, and replication of SARS-associated coronavirus. *The Lancet*, 361:2045-6

Coutinho, M.A.S., Muzitano, M.F., & Costa, S.N.S. (2009). Flavonóides: Potenciais agentes terapêuticos para o processo inflamatório. *Revista Virtual de Química*, 201:241–256.

Dabeek, W.M., and Marra, M.V. (2019, October). Dietary Quercetin and Kaempferol: Bioavailability and Potential Cardiovascular-Related Bioactivity in Humans. *Nutrients*, (10): 2288. DOI: 10.3390/nu11102288

Dai, J.P., Wang, G.F., Li, W.Z., Zhang, L., Yang, J.C., Zhao, X.F.,…Li, K.S. (2012). High-throughput screening for anti-influenza A virus drugs and study of the mechanism of procyanidin on influenza A virus-induced autophagy. *Journal of Biomolecular Screening*, 17, 605–617.

De Costa, F., Yendo, A.C., Fleck, J.D., Gosmann, G., & Fett-Neto, A.G. (2011). Immunoadjuvant and anti-inflammatory plant saponins: characteristics and biotechnological approaches towards sustainable production. *Mini Reviews in Medical Chemistry*, 11 (10) (2011), pp. 857-880.

Dharmananda, S., & Fruehauf, H. *Ginkgo*. (1997). Institute for Traditional Medicine, Portland, Oregon. http://www.itmonline.org/arts/ginkgo.htm

Dharmananda, S. *Shengmai San: An Ancient Formula Now Used in Chinese Hospitals.* (2001). Institute for Traditional Medicine, Portland, Oregon. http://www.itmonline.org/arts/shengmai.htm

Dharmananda, S. *SARS and Chinese Medicine. (2003). How the Chinese People and Institutions Responded with Herbs.* Institute for Traditional Medicine, Portland, Oregon. http://www.itmonline.org/arts/sars.htm

Ding, S., Jiang, H.M., Fang, J. (2018, April). Regulation of Immune Function by Polyphenols. *Journal of Immunology Research.* https://doi.org/10.1155/2018/1264074

Ding, Y., Cao, Z.Y., Cao, L., Ding, G., Wang, Z.Z., & Xiao, W. (2017). Antiviral activity of chlorogenic acid against influenza A (H1N1/H3N2) virus and its inhibition of neuraminidase. *Scientific Report, 7*: 45723

Ding, Y., Zeng, L., Li, R., Chen, Q., Zhou, B., & Chen, Q. (2017). The Chinese prescription lianhuaqingwen capsule exerts anti-influenza activity through the inhibition of viral propagation and impacts immune function. *BMC Complementary and Alternative Medicine.*, 17:130.

Ding, Y.W., Zeng, L.J., Li, R.F., Chen, Q.Y., Zhou, B.X, Chen, Q.L.,...Zhang, F.X. (2017). The Chinese prescription lianhuaqingwen capsule exerts anti-influenza activity through the inhibition of viral propagation and impacts immune function. *BMC Complementary and Alternative Medicine*, 17:130.

Ding, Z., Zhong, R.X., Xi, T.Y., Yang, Y., Xing, N., Wang, W., ...Shu, Z.P. (2020, February). Advances in research into the mechanisms of Chinese Materia Medica against acute lung injury. *Biomedicine & Pharmacotherapy*, Volume 122, 109706.

Dong, L., Xia, J.W., Gong, Y., Chen, Z., Yang, H.H., & Zhang, J. (2014). Effect of Lianhua Qingwen Capsules on Airway Inflammation in Patients with Acute Exacerbation of Chronic Obstructive Pulmonary Disease. *Evidenced Based Complementary and Alternative Medicine*, 1-11.

Dong, Z.L., Lu, X.Y., Tong, X.L., Dong, Y.Q., Tang, L., & Li, M.H. (2017, September). Forsythiae Fructus: A Review on its Phytochemistry, Quality Control, Pharmacology and Pharmacokinetics. *Molecules*, 22(9): 1466. DOI: 10.3390/molecules22091466

Du, C.Y., Zheng, K.Y., Bi, C.W., Dong, T.T., Lin, H., & Tsim, K.W. (2015). Yu Ping Feng San, an Ancient Chinese Herbal Decoction, Induces Gene Expression of Anti-viral Proteins and Inhibits Neuraminidase Activity. *Phytotherapy Research,* 29(5), 656–661. https://doi.org/10.1002/ptr.5290

Du, H.Z., Hou, X.Y., Miao, Y.H., Huang, B.S., & Liu, D.H. (2020). Traditional Chinese Medicine: an effective treatment for 2019 novel coronavirus pneumonia (NCP) [J]. *Chinese Journal of Natural Medicine,* 2020, 18(3): 206-210. DOI: 10.1016/S1875-5364(20)30022-4

Du, J., He, Z.D., Jiang, R.W., Ye, W. C., Xu, H. X., & But, P.P. (2003). Antiviral flavonoids from the root bark of Morus alba L. Phytochemistry, 62(8), 1235–1238. https://doi.org/10.1016/s0031-9422(02)00753-7

Eng, Y.S., Lee, C.H., Lee, W.C., Huang, C.C, & Jung, S.C. (2019). Unraveling the Molecular Mechanism of Traditional Chinese Medicine: Formulas Against Acute Airway Viral Infections as Examples. *Molecules,* 24, 3505;DOI:10.3390/molecules24193505

Efferth, Thomas. (2018, November). Beyond malaria: The inhibition of viruses by artemisinin-type compounds. *Biotechnology Advances,* Volume 36, Issue 6, pp. 1730-1737.

Fei, Y.X., Zhao, B., Yin, Q.Y., Qiu, Y.Y., Ren, G.H., Wang, B.W.,…Li, Y.M. (2019). Ma Xing Shi Gan Decoction attenuates PM2.5 Induced lung Injury via Inhibiting HMGB1/TLR4/NFκB signal pathway in rat. Frontiers in Pharmacology, 10:1361.

Fong, S.Y., Wong, Y.C., Xie, C., & Zuo, Z. (2015). Herb-drug interactions between Scutellariae Radix and mefenamic acid: Simultaneous investigation of pharmacokinetics, anti-inflammatory effect and gastric damage in rats. *Journal of Ethnopharmacology*, 170, 106–116.

Fouad, A., Albuali, W., & Jresat, I. (2016, January). Protective effect of naringenin against lipopolysaccharide-induced acute lung injury in rats. *Pharmacology*.

Fung, K.P., Leung, P.C., Tsui, K.W., Wan, C.C., Wong, K.B., & Waye, M.Y. (2011). Immunomodulatory activities of the herbal formula Kwan Du Bu Fei Tang in healthy subjects: a randomised, double-blind, placebo-controlled study. *Hong Kong Medical Journal*, 17 (Suppl 2):41-3.

Gao, J., Li, J., Shao, X., Jin, Y., Lu, X.W., & Ge, J.F. (2009). Anti-inflammatory and immunoregulatory effects of total glucosides of Yupingfeng powder. *Chinese Medicine Journal* (Engl), 122:1636-41.

Gao, Y., Fang, L., Cai, R.L., Zong, C.J., Chen, X., Lu, J. & Qi, Y. (2014). Shuang-Huang-Lian exerts anti-inflammatory and anti-oxidative activities in lipopolysaccharide-stimulated murine alveolar macrophages. *Phytomedicine*, 21:461-9.

Gao, Y., Fei, Q.L., Qi, R.J., Hou, R., Han, Y.X., Cai, R.L.,…Qi, Y. (2019) Shuang-Huang-Lian Attenuates Airway Hyperresponsiveness and Inflammation in a Shrimp Protein-Induced Murine Asthma Model. *Hindawi Evidence-Based Complementary and Alternative Medicine,* Article ID 4827342, 9 pages. https://doi.org/10.1155/2019/4827342

Ghezzi, P. (2011, January). Role of glutathione in immunity and inflammation in the lung. *International Journal of General Medicine*, 4: 105–113. DOI: 10.2147/IJGM.S15618

Gong, S.J., Su, X.J., Yu, H.P., Li, J., Qin, Y.J., & Xu, Q. (2008). A study on anti-SARS-CoV 3CL protein of flavonoids from litchi chinensis sonn core. *Chinese Pharmacological Bulletin*, 24:699–700.

Gottfried, S. (2109). *The Brain Body Diet*. HarperOne.

Geng, T., Sun, Y., Yao, W., Ding, A., Zhang, L., Guo, J., & Tang, Y. (2011, October). Pharmacokinetics and tissue distribution of schizonepetin in rats. *Fitoterapia*, 82(7):1110-7. DOI: 10.1016/j.fitote.2011.07.008.

Guo, Z.H., Zang, Y.J., & Zhang, L.J. (2019). The efficacy of Polyporus Umbellatus polysaccharide in treating hepatitis B in China. Prog *Molecular Biology and Translational Sciences,* 163:329-360. DOI: 10.1016/bs.pmbts.2019.03.012. Epub 2019 Apr 9.

Grum-Tokars, V., Ratia, K., Begaye, A., Baker, S.C., & Mesecar, A.D. (2008, April). Evaluating the 3C-like protease activity of SARS-Coronavirus: recommendations for standardized assays for drug discovery. *Virus Research*, 133(1):63-73.

Gupta, V., Bansal, P., Singh, R., & Maithani, M. (2010). Herbal antitussives and expectorants - A review. *International Journal of Pharmaceutical Sciences Review and Research*, 5. 5-9.

Hao, D.C., Gu, X.J., Xiao, P.G., & Peng, Y. (2013). Phytochemical and biological research of Fritillaria Medicinal Resources. *Chinese Journal of Natural Medicines,* 11(4):0330-0344. doi:10.3724/SP.J.1009.2013.00330

Hayashi, Y., Matsushima, M., Nakamura, T., Shibasaki, M., Hashimoto, N.; Imaizumi, K.,…Kawabe, T. (2012). Quercetin protects against pulmonary oxidant stress via heme oxygenase-1 induction in lung epithelial cells. *Biochemical and Biophysical Research Communications*, 417, 169–174.

Ho, T.Y., Wu, S.L., Chen, J.C., Li, C.C., & Hsiang C.Y. (2007, May). Emodin blocks the SARS-Coronavirus spike protein and angiotensin-converting enzyme 2 interaction. *Antiviral Research*, 74(2): 92–101. DOI: 10.1016/j..2006.04.014

Ho, T., Wu, S., Chen, J., Li, C., & Hsiang, C. (2007). Emodin blocks the SARS-Coronavirus spike protein and angiotensin-converting enzyme 2 interaction. *Antiviral Research*, 74:92–101.

Hoffmann, M., Kleine-Weber, H., Schroeder, S., Muller, M.A., Drosten, C., & Pohlmann, S. (2020, April). SARS-CoV-2 Cell Entry Depends on ACE2 and TMPRSS2 and Is Blocked by a Clinically Proven Protease Inhibitor. *Cell*, 181, 271–280. *Elsevier Inc.* https://doi.org/10.1016/j.cell.2020.02.052

Horowitz, R.I., Freeman, P.R., & Bruzzese, J. (2020). Efficacy of glutathione therapy in relieving dyspnea associated with COVID-19 pneumonia: A report of 2 cases. Respiratory medicine case reports, 30, 101063. Advance online publication. https://doi.org/10.1016/j.rmcr.2020.101063

Hu, H.W., Xie, X.M., Zhang, P.Z., & Shu, R.G. (2010). (Study on the flavonoids from Mosla chinensis 'jiangxiangru'). *Zhong yao cai = Zhongyaocai Journal of Chinese medicinal materials*, 33. 218-9.

Hu, X., Fu, Y., Lu, X., Zhang, Z., Zhang, W., Cao, Y., & Zhang, N. (2016). Protective effects of platycodin d on lipopolysaccharide-induced acute lung injury by activating LXRalpha-ABCA1 signaling pathway. *Frontiers in Immunology*, 7 (2016), p. 644.

Huang, Y.F., Bai, C., He, F., Xie, Y., & Zhou, H. (2020). Review on the potential action mechanisms of Chinese medicines in treating Coronavirus Disease 2019 (Covid-19). *Pharmacological Research*, 104939. Advance online publication. https://doi.org/10.1016/j.phrs.2020.104939

Huang, X.F., Cheng, W.B., Jiang, Y., Liu, Q., Hong, X., Liu, X.H.,…Huang, H.T. (2020, June). A network pharmacology-based strategy for predicting anti-inflammatory targets of ephedra in treating asthma. *International Immunopharmacology*, Volume 83, 2020, 106423.

Hui, D., Li, S.S., Wu, Q., Jia, K.X., Wu, J., Liu, Y., & Wang, L.S. (2015). Analysis of Active Compounds and Antioxidant Activity Assessment of Six Popular Chinese Juhua Teas. *Natural Product Communications*, Vol 10 No.3 495-498.

Interim Clinical Guidance for Management of Patients with Confirmed Coronavirus Disease (COVID-19). (June 2, 2020). Center for Disease Control and Prevention. https://www.cdc.gov/coronavirus/2019-ncov/hcp/clinical-guidance-management-patients.html#

Imam F., Al-Harbi, N.O., Al-Harbi, M.M., Ansari, M.A., Zoheir, K.M., Iqbal, M.,…Ahmad, S.F. (2015). Diosmin downregulates the expression of T cell receptors, proinflammatory cytokines and NF-κB activation against LPS-induced acute lung injury in mice. *Pharmacology Research*, 102:1–11

Ip, W.K., Chan, K.H., Law, H.K., Tso, G.H., Kong, E.K., Wong, W.H., To, Y.F.,…Lau, Y.L. (2005, May). Mannose-binding lectin in severe acute respiratory syndrome coronavirus infection. *Journal of Infectious Disease*, 15;191(10):1697-704.

Ishitsuka, H., Ohsawa, C., Ohiwa, T., Umeda, I., & Suhara, Y. (1982, October) Antipicornavirus flavone Ro 09-0179. *Antimicrobial Agents and Chemotherapy*, 22(4):611-6.

Ivanescu, B., Miron, A., & Corciova, A. (2015). Sesquiterpene Lactones from Artemisia Genus: Biological Activities and Methods of Analysis. *Journal of Analytical Methods in Chemistry*, 247685. DOI: 10.1155/2015/247685

Jaber, R. (2002). Respiratory and allergic diseases from upper respiratory tract infections to asthma. *Primary Care*, 29(2):231-261.

Jo, S., Kim, S., Shin, D.H., & Kim, M.S. (2020) Inhibition of SARS-CoV 3CL protease by flavonoids. *Journal of Enzyme Inhibition and Medicinal Chemistry*, 35:1, 145-151. DOI: 10.1080/14756366.2019.1690480

Kang, O.H., Chae, H.S., Oh, Y.C., Choi, J.G., Lee, Y.S., Jang, H.J.,…Kwon, D.Y. (2008). Anti-nociceptive and anti-inflammatory effects of Angelicae dahuricae radix through inhibition of the expression of inducible nitric oxide synthase and NO production. *American Journal of Chinese Medicine*, 36(5):913-28.

Kang, O.H., Choi, J.G., Lee, J.H., & Kwon, D.Y. (2010, January). Luteolin Isolated from the Flowers of Lonicera japonica Suppresses Inflammatory Mediator Release by Blocking NF-κB and MAPKs Activation Pathways in HMC-1 Cells. *Molecules,* 15(1), 385-398; https://doi.org/10.3390/molecules15010385

Kao, S.T., Yeh, T.J., Hsieh, C.C., Shiau, H.B., Yeh, Fen, F.T. & Lin, J.G. (2001). The effects of Ma-Xing-Gan-Shi-Tang on respiratory resistance and airway leukocyte infiltration in asthmatic guinea pigs. *Immunopharmacology and Immunotoxicology*, 23. 445-458. 10.1081/IPH-

100107343.

Kun, Wu. (1584). *Yi Fang Kao (Investigations of Medical Formulas)*.

Keyaerts, E., Vijgen, L., Pannecouque, C., Van Damme, E., Peumans, W., Egberink, H., …Van Ranst, M. (2007, September). Plant lectins are potent inhibitors of coronaviruses by interfering with two targets in the viral replication cycle. *Antiviral Research*, 75(3):179-87.

Khaerunnisa, S., Kurniawan, H., Awaluddin, R., Suharta, S., & Soetjipto, S. (2020, March). Potential Inhibitor of Covid-19 Main Protease (Mpro) from Several Medicinal Plant Compounds in Molecular Docking Study. *Preprints.org*. [Epub ahead of print]

Kim, D., Kang, Y.M., Jin, W.Y., Sung, Y., Choi, G., & Kim, H.K. (2014). Antioxidant activities and polyphenol content of Morus alba leaf extracts collected from varying regions. *Biomedical Reports*, 2, 675-680. https://doi.org/10.3892/br.2014.294

Kim, I.S., Park, Y.J., Yoon, S.J., & Lee, H.B. (2010) Ephedrannin A and B from roots of Ephedra Sinica inhibit lipopolysaccharide-induced inflammatory mediators by suppressing nuclear factor-kappaB activation in RAW 264.7 macrophages. *International Immunopharmacology*, 10, 1616–1625.

Kim, H.J., Lee, H.J., Jeong, S.J., Lee, H.J., Kim, S.H., & Park, E.J. (2011). Cortex Mori Radicis extract exerts antiasthmatic effects via enhancement of CD4 + CD 25 + Foxp3 + regulatory T cells and inhibition of Th2 cytokines in a mouse asthma model. *Journal of Ethnopharmacology*, 138, 40–46.10.1016/j.jep.2011.08.021

Kim, M., Seo, K.S., & Yun, K.W. (2018, April). Antimicrobial and Antioxidant Activity of Saposhnikovia divaricata, Peucedanum japonicum and Glehnia littoralis. *The Indian Journal of Pharmaceutical Science*, 80(3):560-565 DOI: 10.4172/pharmaceutical-sciences.1000393

Khachigian, L.M., Collins, T., & Fries, J.W. N-acetyl cysteine blocks mesangial VCAM-1 and NF-kappa B expression in vivo. *American Journal of Pathology*, 1997;151(5):1225–1229.

Kim, A., Im, M., Gu, M.J., & Ma, J.Y. (2016, November). Ethanol extract of Lophatheri Herba exhibits anti-cancer activity in human cancer cells by suppression of metastatic and angiogenic potential. *Science Reports*, 3;6:36277. DOI: 10.1038/srep36277.

Kong, D.Z., Liang, N., Liu, J.P., Nikolova, D., Jakobsen, J.C., & Gluud, C. (2018, August). Xiao Chai Hu Tang, a Chinese herbal medicine formula, for chronic hepatitis B. *Cochrane Database of Systematic Review*, (8):CD013090.DOI: 10.1002/14651858.CD013090

Kuo, M.Y., Liao, M.F., Chen, F.L., Li, Y.C., Yang, M.L., Lin, R.H., & Kuan, Y.H. (2011). Luteolin attenuates the pulmonary inflammatory response involves abilities of antioxidation and inhibition of MAPK and NFkappaB pathways in mice with endotoxin-induced acute lung injury. *Food Chemistry and Toxicology, 49*, 2660–2666.

Lago, J.H.G., Toledo-Arruda, A.C., Mernak, M., Barrosa, K.H., Martins, M.A., Tibério L.F.L.C., & Prado C.M. (2014). Structure-Activity Association of Flavonoids in Lung Diseases. *Brazil Molecules,* 19(3), 3570-3595; https://doi.org/10.3390/molecules19033570

Lau, J.T., Leung, P.C, Wong, E.L.Y., Fong, C., Cheng, K.F., Zhang, S.C.,...Ko, W.M. (2005). The use of an herbal formula by hospital care workers during the severe acute respiratory syndrome epidemic in Hong Kong to prevent severe acute respiratory syndrome transmission, relieve influenza-related symptoms, and improve quality of life: a prospective cohort study. *Journal of Alternative and Complementary Medicine*, 11:49-55.

Lau, K.M., Lee, K.M., Koon, C.M., Cheung, C.S., Lau, C.P., Ho, H.M.,...Fung, K.P. (2008, June). Immunomodulatory and anti-SARS activities of Houttuynia Cordata. *Journal of Ethnopharmacology*, 118(1):79-85. DOI: 10.1016/j.jep.2008.03.018

Lau, L. (2020, March). *New Coronavirus Disease Diagnosis and Treatment Plan: Interim 7th Edition March 3, 2020*. Extract translated from the People's Republic of China State Council official website by Lawrence Lau, L.Ac, Senior Practitioner at Yo San University of Traditional Chinese Medicine. www.yosan.edu. http://www.gov.cn/zhengce/zhengceku/2020-03/04/content_5486705.htm

Law, H.Y., Yang, L.H., Lau, S.Y., & Chan, G.C. (2017). Antiviral effect of forsythoside A from Forsythia suspensa (Thunb.) Vahl fruit against influenza A virus through reduction of viral M1 protein. *Journal of Ethnopharmacology*, 209: 236-247.

Lee, D.S., Boo, K.H., & Kim, Y.C. (2014, April). The Effects of Areca catechu L. Extract. *Korean Journal of Food Science and Technology*, 46(2):245-248. DOI: 10.9721/KJFST.2014.46.2.245

Lem, F.F., Opook, F., Herng, D.L.J., Na, C.S., Lawson, F.P., & Tyng, C.F. (2020, April). Molecular mechanism of action of repurposed drugs and traditional Chinese medicine used for the treatment of patients infected with Covid-19: A systematic scoping review. *MedRxiv* preprint, DOI: https://doi.org/10.1101/2020.0 4.10.20060376.

Lewicki, S., Skopińska-Różewska, E., Brewczyńska, A, & Zdanowski, R. (2017, October). Administration of Rhodiola kirilowii Extracts during Mouse Pregnancy and Lactation Stimulates Innate but Not Adaptive Immunity of the Offspring. *Journal of Immunological Research*, DOI: 10.1155/2017/8081642

Li, C.W., Chen, Z.W., Wu, X.L., Ning, Z.X., Su, Z.Q., Li, Y.C., & Lai, X.P. (2015, March). A Standardized Traditional Chinese Medicine Preparation Named Yejuhua Capsule Ameliorates Lipopolysaccharide-Induced Acute Lung Injury in Mice via Downregulating Toll-Like Receptor 4/Nuclear Factor- κ B. *Evidence-Based Complementary and Alternative Medicine*, 264612. 10.1155/2015/264612.

Li, W., Zhao, R., Wang, X., Liu, F., Zhao, J., Yao, Q.,…Niu, X. (2018). Nobiletin-ameliorated lipopolysaccharide-induced inflammation in acute lung injury by suppression of NF-kappaB pathway in vivo and vitro. *Inflammation*, 41 (3), pp. 996-1007.

Li, R.F., Ho, Y.L., Huang, J.C., Pan, W.X., Ma, Q.H., Shi, Y.X.,…Yang, Z.F. (2020, June). Lianhuaqingwen exerts anti-viral and anti-inflammatory activity against novel coronavirus (SARS-CoV-2). *Pharmacological Research,* Volume 156, 104761.

Li, X., Lin, J., Han, W., Mai, W., Wang, L., Li, Q.,…Chen, D. (2012). Antioxidant ability and mechanism of rhizoma Atractylodes macrocephala. *Molecules* (Basel, Switzerland), 17(11), 13457–13472. https://doi.org/10.3390/molecules171113457

Li, X.W., Genga, M.M., Peng, Y.Z., Meng, L.S., & Lua, S.M. (2020, April). Molecular immune pathogenesis and diagnosis of Covid-19. *Journal of Pharmaceutical Analysis*, Volume 10, Issue 2, pp. 102-108. https://doi.org/10.1016/j.jpha.2020.03.001

Li, Z.X., Zhao, G.D., & Xiong, W. (2019). Immunomodulatory effects of a new whole ingredients extract from Astragalus: a combined evaluation on chemistry and pharmacology. *Chinese Medicine*, 14, 12. https://doi.org/10.1186/s13020-019-0234-0

Lin, C.W., Tsai, F.J., Tsai, C.H., Lai, C.C., Wan, L., Ho, T.Y.,...Chao, P.D. (2005, October). Anti-SARS-Coronavirus 3C-like protease effects of Isatis indigotica root and plant-derived phenolic compounds. *Antiviral Research*, 68(1):36-42.

Lin, Y.N., Zhu, D.N, Qi, J., Qin, M.J., & Yu, B.Y. (2010, September). Characterization of homoisoflavonoids in different cultivation regions of Ophiopogon japonicus and related antioxidant activity. *Journal of Pharmaceutical and Biomedical Analysis*, 5; 52(5):757-62.

Lindequist, U., Lesnau, A., Teuscher, E., & Pilgrim, H. (1989). Antiviral activity of ergosterol peroxide. *Pharmazie*, 44:579–80.

Liu, J., McIntosh, H., & Lin, H. (2001). Chinese medicinal herbs for chronic hepatitis B: a systematic review. *Liver*, 21(4), 280–286. https://doi.org/10.1034/j.1600-0676.2001.021004280.x

Liu, X.X., Yu, D.D., Chen, M.J., Sun, T., Li, G., Huang, W.J.,…Ren, B.X. (2015). Hesperidin ameliorates lipopolysaccharide-induced acute lung injury in mice by inhibiting HMGB1 release. *International immunopharmacology*, 25(2), 370–376. https://doi.org/10.1016/j.intimp.2015.02.022

Liu, Y., Jing, Y.Y., & Zeng, C.Y. (2018, January). Scutellarin suppresses NLRP3 Inflammasome activation in macrophages and protects mice against bacterial sepsis. *Frontiers in Pharmacology*, 8:975. DOI:10.3389/fphar.2017.00975

Liu, Z., Zhong, J. Y., Gao, E. N., & Yang, H. (2014). Effects of glycyrrhizin acid and licorice flavonoids on LPS-induced cytokines expression in macrophage. *Zhongguo Zhong yao za zhi = Zhongguo zhongyao zazhi = China journal of Chinese Materia Medica*, 39(19), 3841–3845.

Louati, S., Simmonds, M., Grayer, R., Kite, G., & Mohamed, D. (2003). Flavonoids from Eriobotrya japonica (Rosaceae) growing in Tunisia. *Biochemical Systematics and Ecology*, 31. 99-101. 10.1016/S0305-1978(02)00072-8.

Lu, Y., Jiang, J., Ling, L.J., Zhang, Y.Y., Li, H., & Chen, D.F. (2018). Beneficial effects of Houttuynia Cordata polysaccharides on "two-hit" acute lung injury and endotoxic fever in rats associated with anti-complementary activities. *Acta Pharmaceutica Sinica B*. https://doi.org/10.1016/j.apsb.2017.11.003

Lu, W., Zheng, B.J., Xu, K., Schwarz, W., Du, L., Wong, C.K.,…Sun, B. (2006, August). Severe acute respiratory syndrome-associated coronavirus 3a protein forms an ion channel and modulates virus release. *Proceedings of the National Academy of Sciences U S A*, 15; 103(33):12540-5.

Luo, W.S., Su, X.J., Gong, S.J., Qin, Y.J., Liu, W.B., Li, J.,…Xu, Q. (2009). Anti-SARS-Coronavirus 3C-like protease effects of Rheum Palmatum L. extracts. *BioScience Trends*, 3(4):124-126.

Luo, H., Tang, Q.L., Shang, Y.X., Liang, S.B., Yang, M., Robinson, N., & Liu, J.P. (2020, April). Can Chinese Medicine Be Used for Prevention of CoronaVirus Disease 2019 (Covid-19)? A Review of Historical Classics, Research Evidence and Current Prevention Programs. *Chinese Journal of Integrative Medicine*, 26(4):243-250. DOI: 10.1007/s11655-020-3192-6

Ma, N.H., Guo, J., Chen, S.H.X., Yuan, X.R., Zhang, T., & Ding, Y. (2020, January). Antioxidant and Compositional HPLC Analysis of Three Common Bamboo Leaves. *Molecules,* 25(2), 409; https://doi.org/10.3390/molecules25020409

Middleton, E., & Kandaswami, C. (1992). Effects of flavonoids on immune and inflammatory cell functions. *Biochemical Pharmacology*, 43, 1167–1179.

Miean, K.H. & Mohamed, S. (2001). Flavonoid (Myricetin, Quercetin, Kaempferol, Luteolin, and Apigenin) Content of Edible Tropical Plants. *Journal of Agricultural and Food Chemistry,* 49 (6), 3106-3112, DOI: 10.1021/jf000892m

Mijnhout, G. (2010, April). Natural Standard Patient Monograph, "Alpha-lipoic acid." *The Netherlands Journal of Medicine*, vol 68: pp 158-160.

Min, Wu. *(1530). Fu Shou Jing Fang* (Exquisite Formulas for Fostering Longevity). n.p.

Miyagoshi, M., Amagaya, S., & Ogihara, Y. (1986) Antitussive effects of L-ephedrine, amygdalin, and makyokansekito (Chinese traditional medicine) using a cough model induced by sulfur dioxide gas in mice. *Planta Medica*, 4, 275–278.

National Health Commission. Press conference of the joint prevention and control mechanism of the State Council on. http://www.nhc.gov.cn/xcs/fkdt/202004/05f7318e9fb84b419b35559bc02a42f4.shtml. Referenced from *The Lancet.* https://www.thelancet.com/journals/lancet/article/PIIS0140-6736(20)31143-0/fulltext

National Institute of Health Treatment Guidelines. What's New in the Guidelines. (June 16, 2020). https://www.covid19treatmentguidelines.nih.gov/whats-new/

Neuman, M.G., Cohen, L.B., Opris, M., Nanau, R., & Hyunjin, J. (2015). Hepatotoxicity of Pyrrolizidine Alkaloids. *Journal of Pharmacy and Pharmacological Science*, 18(4) 825-843.

Ngan, L.T., Jang, M.J., Kwon, M.J., & Ahn, Y.J. (2015). Antiviral activity and possible mechanism of action of constituents identified in Paeonia lactiflora root toward human rhinoviruses. *PLoS ONE*, 10, e0121629.

Nguyen, T.T., Woo, H.J., Kang, H.K., Nguyen, V.D., Kim, Y.M., Kim, D.W.,...Kim, D. (2012, May). Flavonoid-mediated inhibition of SARS coronavirus 3C-like protease expressed in Pichia pastoris. *Biotechnology Letters*, 34(5), 831–838. https://doi.org/10.1007/s10529-011-0845-8

Niu, M., Wang, R.L., Wang, Z.X., Zhang, P., Bai, Z.F., Jing, J.,... Xiao, X.H. (2020, March). Rapid establishment of traditional Chinese medicine prevention and treatment of 2019-nCoV based on clinical experience and molecular docking. *Zhongguo Zhong Yao Za Zhi*, 45(6):1213-1218. DOI: 10.19540/j.cnki.cjcmm.20200206.501.

Ozçelik, B., Gürbüz, I., Karaoglu, T., & Yeşilada, E. (2009). Antiviral and antimicrobial activities of three sesquiterpene lactones from Centaurea solstitialis L. ssp. solstitialis. *Microbiological Research*, 164:545–552. 2009.

Pal, M., Berhanu, G., Desalegn, C., & Kandi, V. (2020). Severe Acute Respiratory Syndrome Coronavirus-2 (SARS-CoV-2): An Update. *Cureus*, 12(3), e7423. https://doi.org/10.7759/cureus.7423

Park, J.Y., Kim, J.H., Kim, Y.M., Jeong, H.J., Kim, D.W.,…Park, K.H. (2012). Tanshinones as selective and slow-binding inhibitors for SARS-CoV cysteine proteases. Bioorganic and Medicinal Chemistry 20, pp. 5928-5935.

Patel, V.J., Biswas, R., Mehta, H.J., Joo, M., & Sadikot, R.T. (2018). Alternative and natural therapies for acute lung injury and acute respiratory distress syndrome. *BioMed Research International*, Article 2476824.

Peng, M., Watanabe, S., Chan, K.W.K., He, Q., Zhao, Y., Zhang, Z.,…Li G (2017, July). Luteolin restricts dengue virus replication through inhibition of the proprotein convertase furin. *Antiviral Research*, 143:176-185. DOI: 10.1016/j..2017.03.026.

Peng, W. J., Xin, R. H., Luo, Y. J., Liang, G., Ren, L. H., Liu, Y.,…Zheng, J. F. (2016). Evaluation of the acute and subchronic toxicity of Aster tataricus L.F. *African Journal of Complementary and Alternative Medicine*, 13(6), 38–53.

Phurimsak, C., & Leardkamolkarn, V. (2005). Screening for antiviral effect of Thai herbs; Kaempferia parviflora, Ellipeiopsis cherrevensis and Stemona tuberosa against Dengue virus type-2. *31st Congress on Science and Technology of Thailand.* Suranaree University of Technology.

Rafi, M., Devi, A.F., & Syafitri, U.D. (2020). Classification of Andrographis paniculata extracts by solvent extraction using HPLC fingerprint and chemometric analysis. *BMC Research Notes*, 13, 56. https://doi.org/10.1186/s13104-020-4920-x

Rahman A., Fazal F. (2011). Blocking NF-κB. *Proceedings of The American Thoracic Society*, 8(6):497–503. DOI: 10.1513/pats.201101-009MW.

Rajgopal, A., Missler, S. R., & Scholten, J. D. (2016). Magnolia officinalis (Hou Po) bark extract stimulates the Nrf2-pathway in hepatocytes and protects against oxidative stress. *Journal of Ethnopharmacology*, 193, 657–662. https://doi.org/10.1016/j.jep.2016.10.016

Reddy, A.M., Seo, J.H., Ryu, S.Y., Kim, Y.S., Kim, Y.S., Min, K.R., & Kim, Y. (2004). Cinnamaldehyde and 2-methoxycinnamaldehyde as NF-kappaB inhibitors from Cinnamomum cassia. *Planta Medica*, 70, 823–827.

Santangelo, C., Varì, R., Scazzocchio, B., Di Benedetto, R., Filesi, C., & Masella, R. (2007). Polyphenols, intracellular signalling and inflammation. *Annali Dell'Istituto Superiore Di Sanita*, 43(4), 394–405.

Sahoo, M., Jena, L., Rath, S.N., & Kumar, S. (2016). Identification of Suitable Natural Inhibitor against Influenza A (H1N1) Neuraminidase Protein by Molecular Docking. *Genomics and Informatics*, 14, 96–103.

Schwarz, S., Wang, K., Yu, W.J., Sun, B., & Schwarz, W. (2011). Emodin inhibits current through SARS-associated coronavirus 3a protein. *Antiviral Research*, 90:64-9.

Schwarz, S., Sauter, D., Wang, K., Zhang, R.H., Sun, B., Karioti, A.,… Schwarz, W. (2014, February). Kaempferol Derivatives as antiviral drugs against the 3a Channel Protein of Coronavirus. *Planta Medica*, 80(02-03): 177–182. DOI: 10.1055/s-0033-1360277

Shi, L.H., Yin, F.L., Xin, X.G., Mao, S.M., Hu, P.P, Zhao, C.Z., & Sun, X.N. (2014). Astragalus Polysaccharide Protects Astrocytes from Being Infected by HSV-1 through TLR3/NF-κB Signaling Pathway. *Evidence Based Complementary and Alternative Medicine*, 285356. https://doi.org/10.1002/bmc.3055

Shi, X.B., Sun, H.Z., Zhou, D., Xi, H.J., & Shan, L.N. (2015). Arctigenin attenuates lipopolysaccharide-induced acute lung injury in rats. *Inflammation*, 38 (2), pp. 623-631.

Song, W., Si, L., Ji, S., Wang, H., Fang, X.M., Yu, L.Y.,…Ye, M.(2014). Uralsaponins M-Y, triterpenoid saponins from the roots of Radix Glycyrrhizae. *Journal of Natural Products*, 77, 1632–1643.

Spagnolo, P., Balestro E., Aliberti, S., Cocconcelli, E., Biondini, D., Casaet, G.,…Maher, T. (2020, May). Pulmonary fibrosis secondary to COVID-19: a call to arms? *The Lancet, Respiratory Medicine*. DOI:https://doi.org/10.1016/S2213-2600(20)30222-8

Su, X.D., Jang, H., Li, H.X., Kim, Y.H., & Yang, S.Y. (2019, November). Identification of potential inflammatory inhibitors from Aster tataricus. *Bioorganic Chemistry*, 92:103208. DOI: 10.1016/j.bioorg.2019.103208.

Suzuki, Y.J., Aggarwal, B.B., & Packer, L. (1992) Alpha-lipoic acid is a potent inhibitor of NF-kappa B activation in human T cells. *Biochemistry and*

Biophysics Research Communications, 189(3):1709–1715. DOI: 10.1016/0006-291x(92)90275-p.

Taiping Huimin Pharmaceutical Bureau. (1078). *Tai Ping Hui Min He Ji Ju Fang* (Imperial Grace Formulary of the Tai Ping Era).

Takahashi, S., Yoshiya, T., Yoshizawa-Kumagaye, K., & Sugiyama, T. (2015). Nicotianamine is a novel angiotensin-converting enzyme 2 inhibitor in soybean. *Biomedical Research*, 36(3):219-24. DOI: 10.2220/biomedres.36.219

Tan, Z.H., Y, L.H., Wei, H.L., & Liu, G.T. (2009, September) Scutellarin protects against lipopolysaccharide-induced acute lung injury via inhibition of NF-κB activation in mice. *Journal of Asian Natural Products Research*, 12:3, pp. 175- 184. https://doi.org/10.1080/10286020903347906

Tang, W. *(1798). Wen Bing Tiao Bian* (Systematic Differentiation of Warm Disease). n.p.

Tao, W., Su, Q., Wang, H., Guo, S., Chen, Y., Duan, J., & Wang, S. (2015). Platycodin D attenuates acute lung injury by suppressing apoptosis and inflammation in vivo and in vitro. *International Immunopharmacology*, 27 (1) pp. 138-147.

The People's Republic of China National Health Commission, Office of the National Administration of Traditional Chinese Medicine. Administrative Notice 2020 (22). "*Notice on Recommending the Use of Qing Fei Bai Du Tang in the Integrated Traditional Chinese and Western Medicine Treatment of Pneumonia Caused by the New Coronavirus*". Source: People's Republic of China, State Council Official Website (in Chinese).

http://www.gov.cn/zhengce/zhengceku/2020-03/04/content_5486705.htm

The State Council, The People's Republic of China. *Latest developments in epidemic control 17 February 2020*. The State Council, The People's Republic of China, 2020.

Thiel, V., Ivanov, K.A., Putics, A., Hertzig, T., Schelle, B., Bayer, S.,…Ziebuhr, J. (2003, September). Mechanisms and enzymes involved in SARS coronavirus genome expression. *Journal of General Virology*, 84:2305-15.

Tian, H., Liu, Z.J., Pu, Y.W., & Bao, Y.X. (2019, April). Immunomodulatory effects exerted by Poria Cocos polysaccharides via TLR4/TRAF6/NF-κB signaling in vitro and in vivo. *Biomedicine and Pharmacotherapy*, 112:108709. DOI:10.1016/j.biopha.2019.108709.

Tian, X., Cheng, Z.Y., Jin, H., Gao, J., & Qiao, H.L. (2013). Inhibitory Effects of Baicalin on the Expression and Activity of CYP3A Induce the Pharmacokinetic Changes of Midazolam in Rats. *Evidence Based Complementary and Alternative Medicine*, 179643.

Tibullo, D., Li Volti, G., & Giallongo, C. (2017). Biochemical and clinical relevance of alpha lipoic acid: antioxidant and anti-inflammatory activity, molecular pathways and therapeutic potential. *Inflammation Research*, 66:947-959.

Traditional Medicine Research. (2020). Evidence Bridging Science and Tradition.
https://www.tmrjournals.com/tmr/EN/subject/listSubjectArticle.do?subjectId=1552545879963#

United States Foods and Drug Administration. (2020). *Covid-19 Frequently Asked Questions.* https://www.fda.gov/emergency-preparedness-and-response/coronavirus-disease-2019-covid-19/covid-19-frequently-asked-questions

Wang, C.T., Li, Q.T. & Li, T.Y. (2020). Dioscin alleviates lipopolysaccharide-induced acute lung injury through suppression of TLR4 signaling pathways. *Experimental Lung Research*, 46:1-2, 11-22, DOI: 10.1080/01902148.2020.1711830

Wang, J., Zhang, T.Z., Ma, C.H., & Wang, S.M. (2015). Puerarin attenuates airway inflammation by regulation of eotaxin-3. *Immunology Letters*, 163, pp. 173–178.

Wang, K., Xie, S.Q., & Sun, B. (2011, February). Viral proteins function as ion channels. *Biochimica et Biophysica Acta*, 1808(2):510-5.

Wang, P.H. (2008). Toona Sinensis Roem (Meliaceae) leaf extract alleviates hyperglycemia via altering adipose glucose transporter 4. *Food and Chemical Toxicology*, 46, pp. 2554-2560.

Wang, Q.H., Wong, G., Lu, G.W., Yan, J.H., & Gao, G. F. (2016). MERS-CoV spike protein: targets for vaccines and therapeutics. *Antiviral Research*, 133, pp. 165–177.

Wang, W.J., Ma, X.T., Han, J.C., Zhou, M.J., Ren, H.H., Pan, Q.W.,...Zheng Q.S. (2016, January). Neuroprotective Effect of Scutellarin on Ischemic Cerebral Injury by Down-Regulating the Expression of Angiotensin-Converting Enzyme and AT1 Receptor. *PLoS One*, 11(1):e0146197. DOI: 10.1371/journal.pone.0146197.

Wang, X.G., & Liu, Z.J. (2014). Prevention and treatment of viral respiratory infections by traditional Chinese herbs. *Chinese Medicine Journal* (Engl), 127(7):1344-50.

Wang, X.T., Yan, J.J., Xu, X.H., Duan, C.Y., Xie, Z., Ma, H.X.,...Du, X.C. (2018, May). Puerarin prevents LPS-induced acute lung injury via inhibiting inflammatory response. *Microbial Pathogenesis,* 118:170-176. DOI: 10.1016/j.micpath.2018.03.033.

Wang, Y., Liu, Y., Zhang, X.Y., Xu, L.H., Ouyang, D.Y., Liu, K.P.,...He, X.H. (2014, November). Ginsenoside Rg1 regulates innate immune responses in macrophages through differentially modulating the NF-κB and PI3K/Akt/mTOR pathways. *International Immunopharmacology,* 23(1):77-84.

World Health Organization. *Modes of transmission of virus causing COVID-19: implications for IPC precaution recommendations. Scientific brief.* (March 29, 2020). Geneva: World Health Organization; 2020. https://www.who.int/news-room/commentaries/detail/modes-of-transmission-of-virus-causing-covid-19-implications-for-ipc-precaution-recommendations

Wu, C.M., Chen, X.Y, Cai, Y.P., Xia, J.A., Zhou, X., Xu, S.,...Song, Y.L. (2020). Risk Factors Associated With Acute Respiratory Distress Syndrome and Death in Patients With Coronavirus Disease 2019 Pneumonia in Wuhan, China. *JAMA internal medicine,* e200994. Advance online publication. https://doi.org/10.1001/jamainternmed.2020.0994

Wu, C.R., Yang, L., Yang, Y.Y., Zhang, P., Zhong, W., Wang, Y.L.,...Li, H. (2020, February) Analysis of therapeutic targets for SARS-CoV-2 and discovery of potential drugs by computational method. *Acta Pharmaceutica Sinica B.* https://doi.org/10.1016/j.apsb.2020.02.008

Wu, C.Y., Jan, J.T., Ma, S.H., Kuo, C.J., Juan, H.F., Cheng, Y.S.E.,...Wong, C.H. (2004, July). Small molecules targeting severe acute respiratory syndrome human coronavirus. *Proceedings of the National Academy of Sciences*, 101 (27) 10012-10017; DOI: 10.1073/pnas.0403596101

Wu, H.H., Wang, J.Q., Yang, Y.W., Li, T.Y., Cao, Y.J., Qu, Y.X.,...Sun, Y.K. (2020). Preliminary exploration of the mechanism of Qing Fei Pai Du decoction against novel coronavirus pneumonia based on network pharmacology and molecular docking technology, *Acta Pharmaceutica Sinica*. DOI: 10.16438/j.0513-4870.2020-0136.

Xia, S.A., Liu, Q., Wang, Q., Sun, Z.W., Su, S., Du, L.Y.,...Jiang, S.B. (2014). Middle East respiratory syndrome coronavirus (MERS-CoV) entry inhibitors targeting spike protein. *Virus Research*, 194, pp. 200-210.

Xiao, Y.C., Olatunde, O.Z., & Yong, J.P. (2020). Progress of chemical components and biological activities of Fructus Amomi. *Archives of Biotechnology and Biomedicine*, 5:001-004.

Xu, Z.R., Kun, Li., Pan, T.W., Liu, J., Bin, Li., Li, C.X.,...Liu, X.G. (2019, July). Lonicerin, an anti-algE flavonoid against Pseudomonas aeruginosa virulence screened from Shuanghuanglian formula by molecule docking based strategy. *Journal of Ethnopharmacology,* Volume 239, 111909. https://doi.org/10.1016/j.jep.2019.111909

Yang, Q.S., He, L.P., Zhou, X.L., Zhao, Y., Shen, J., Xu, P., & Ni, S.Z. (2015) Kaempferol pretreatment modulates systemic inflammation and oxidative stress following hemorrhagic shock in mice. *Chinese Medicine*, 10:6.

Yang, R.C., Liu, H., Bai, C., Wang, Y.C., Zhang, X.H., Guo, R.,...& Wang, Y. (2020). Chemical composition and pharmacological mechanism of Qingfei Paidu Decoction and Ma Xing Shi Gan Decoction against Coronavirus Disease 2019 (COVID-19): In silico and experimental study. *Pharmacological Research*, 157, 104820. Advance online publication. https://doi.org/10.1016/j.phrs.2020.104820

Yang, X.Z., Zhu, J.Y., Tang, C.P., Ke, C.Q., Lin, G., Cheng, T.Y.,... & Ye, Y. (2008). Alkaloids from Roots of Stemona sessilifolia and Their Antitussive Activities. *Planta Medica*, 75. 174-7. 10.1055/s-0028-1088345.

Yang, Y., Islam, S., Wang, J., Li, Y., & Chen, X. (2020 *International Journal of Biological Sciences*, 16(10): 1708–1717. DOI: 10.7150/ijbs.45538

Yang, Y.R., Huang, Y., Huang, C., Lv, X.W., Liu, L.P., Wang, Y.Y., & Li, J. (2012, December). Antifibrosis effects of triterpene acids of Eriobotrya japonica (Thunb.) Lindl. leaf in a rat model of bleomycin-induced pulmonary fibrosis. *Journal of Pharmacy and Pharmacology*, 64(12):1751-60. DOI: 10.1111/j.2042-7158.2012.01550.x.

Yi, L., Li, Z.G., Yuan, K.H., Qu, X.X., Chen, J., Wang, G.W.,... Xia, X.J. (2004). Small molecules blocking the entry of severe acute respiratory syndrome coronavirus into host cells. *Journal of Virology*, 78:11334-9.

Yin, X.L., Chen, L., Liu, Y., Yang, J.L., Ma, C.Q, Yao, Z.Y.,...Li, M.Y. (2010). Enhancement of the innate immune response of bladder epithelial cells by Astragalus polysaccharides through upregulation of TLR4 expression. *Biochemical and Biophysical Research Communications*, 397(2):232–8.

Ying, T. (2020). Specific Applications of Traditional Chinese Medicine (TCM) in the Prevention and Treatment of COVID-19 (2019-nCoV) & Integration of TCM into Educational Curriculum. Compiled, Translated and written by Lori Hsu, MTOM, & Debra Nash-Galpern, L.Ac., DiplOM Editors: Donna Chow, L.Ac., DiplOM. https://www.elotus.org/promo-files/COVID-19_resources/eLotus%20Article%202%20Covid%2019%20English.pdf

Yoon, J. H., & Baek, S. J. (2005). Molecular targets of dietary polyphenols with anti-inflammatory properties. *Yonsei Medical Journal*, 46(5), 585–596. https://doi.org/10.3349/ymj.2005.46.5.585

Yu, H., Qiu, J.F., Ma, L.J., Hu, Y.J., Li, P., & Wan, J.B. (2017, October) Phytochemical and phytopharmacological review of Perilla frutescens L. (Labiatae), a traditional edible-medicinal herb in *China Food and Chemical Toxicology*, Volume 108, Part B, pp. 375-391.

Yu, H.L., Zhao, T.F., Wu, H., Pan, Y.Z., Zhang, Q., Wang, K.L.,… Jin, Y.P. (2015). Pinellia ternata lectin exerts a proinflammatory effect on macrophages by inducing the release of proinflammatory cytokines, the activation of the nuclear factor-kappaB signaling pathway and the overproduction of reactive oxygen species. *International Journal of Molecular Medicine*, 36, 1127–1135.

Yu, M.S., Lee, J., Lee, J.M., Kim, Y., Chin, Y.W. & Jee, J.G. (2012). Identification of myricetin and scutellarein as novel chemical inhibitors of the SARS-Coronavirus helicase, nsP13. *Bioorganic and Medicinal Chemistry Letters*, 22:4049-54

Yu, Y., Zhu, C.G., Wang, S.J, Song, W.X., Yang, Y.C., & Shi, J.G. (2013). Homosecoiridoid alkaloids with amino acid units from the flower buds of Lonicera japonica. *Journal of Natural Products*, 76(12), 2226–2233. https://doi.org/10.1021/np4005773

Yuan, L.D. (1247). *Nei Wai Shang Bian Huo Luo* (Clarification about Internal and External Disease Causation). n.p.

Yun, M.Y., & Yi, Y.S. (2019). Regulatory roles of ginseng on inflammatory caspases, executioners of inflammasome activation. *Journal of Ginseng Research*. 44. 10.1016/j.jgr.2019.12.006.

Zakaryan, H., Arabyan, E., Oo, A., & Zandi, K. (2017, September). Flavonoids: promising natural compounds against viral infections. *Archives of Virology*, 162(9):2539-2551.

Zhang, L.L, Xu, W., Xu, Y.L., Chen, X., Huang, M., & Lu, J.J. (2017, August). Therapeutic potential of Rhizoma Alismatis: a review on ethnomedicinal application, phytochemistry, pharmacology, and toxicology. *Annals of The New York Academy of Sciences*, 1401(1):90-101. DOI: 10.1111/nyas.13381.

Zhang, B.M., Wang, Z.B., Xin, P., Wang, Q.H., Bu, H., & Kuang, H.X. (2018). Phytochemistry and pharmacology of genus Ephedra. *Chinese Journal of Natural Medicine*, 16, 811–828.

Zhang, A., Pan, W.Y., Lv, J., & Wu, H. (2017). Protective effect of amygdalin on LPS-induced acute lung injury by inhibiting NF-kappaB and NLRP3 signaling pathways. *Inflammation*, 40 (3) (2017), pp. 745-751.

Zhang, D.H., Wu, K.L., Zhang, X., Deng, S.Q., & Peng, B. (2020, February). In silico screening of Chinese herbal medicines with the potential to directly inhibit 2019 novel coronavirus. *Journal of Integrative Medicine.* DOI: 10.1016/j.joim.2020.02.005

Zhang, D., Li, S., Wang, N., Tan, H. Y., Zhang, Z., & Feng, Y. (2020). The Cross-Talk Between Gut Microbiota and Lungs in Common Lung Diseases. *Frontiers in Microbiology*, 11, 301. https://doi.org/10.3389/fmicb.2020.00301

Zhang, L.W., Ji, T., Su, S. L., Shang, E. X., Guo, S., Guo, J. M.,…Duan, J. A. (2017). Pharmacokinetics of Mori Folium Flavones and Alkaloids in Normal and Diabetic Rats. *Zhongguo Zhong yao za zhi = Zhongguo zhongyao zazhi = China journal of Chinese materia medica*, 42(21), 4218–4225. https://doi.org/10.19540/j.cnki.cjcmm.20170901.008

Zhang, Y.S., Wang, Z.M., Zhu, J.L., Chen, B., & Li, Y.J. (2012). Determination of atractylodin in rat plasma by HPLC-UV method and its application to a Pharmacokinetic study. *Journal of Liquid Chromatography and Related Technologies,* 35:778–787. DOI: 10.1080/10826076.2011.608235.

Zhang, Z.J., Mitchell, C., Wiseman, N., & Ye, Feng. (200 AD and republished in 1998). In: *Shang Han Lun, On Cold Damage, Translation, and Commentaries.* Paradigm Publications.

Zhang, Z.J., Wilms, S., & Wiseman, N. (200 CE and republished in 2013). In: *Jin Gui Yao Lue: Essential Prescriptions of the Golden Cabinet, Translation & Commentaries.* Paradigm Publications.

Zhao, D.X., Hu, B.Q., Zhang, M., Zhang, C.F., & Xu, X.H. (2014, December). Simultaneous separation and determination of phenolic acids, pentapeptides, and triterpenoid saponins in the root of Aster tataricus by high-performance liquid chromatography coupled with electrospray ionization quadrupole time-of-flight mass spectrometry. https://doi.org/10.1002/jssc.201401008

Zhao, J.S. Tian, S., Yang, J., Liu, J.F., & Zhang, W. (2020). Investigating the mechanism of Qing-Fei-Pai-Du- Tang for the treatment of novel coronavirus pneumonia by network pharmacology. *Chinese Traditional and Herbal Drugs.*
http://kns.cnki.net/kcms/detail/12.1108.R.20200216.2044.002.html.

Zheng, Y.H. (2010). Investigation of prescription to treat influenza A virus subtype H1N1 in Beijing Youan hospital. *Shanxi Medical Journal,* 39: 897-898.

Zhi, H.J., Zhu, H.Y., Zhang, Y.Y., Lu, Y., Li, H., & Chen, D.F. (2019). In vivo effect of quantified flavonoids-enriched extract of Scutellaria baicalensis root on acute lung injury induced by influenza A virus. *Phytomedicine,* 57, pp. 105-116

Zhou, J.H., Wu, W.P., Xie, Z.M., & Sun, W.J. (2004). Studies on the fingerprint and quantitative analysis of quercetin from Aster tataricus. *Zhong yao cai = Zhongyaocai = Journal of Chinese medicinal materials,* 27(8), 562–565.

Zhou, L.J., Liu, Z.J., Wang, Z.X., Yu, S., Long, T.T., Zhou, X., & Bao, Y.X. (2017). Astragalus polysaccharides exert immunomodulatory effects via TLR4-mediated MyD88-dependent signaling pathway in vitro and in vivo. *Scientific Reports,* volume 7, article number: 44822.

Zhou, P., Yang, X.L., Wang, X.F., Hu, B., Zhang, l., Zhang, W.,…Zheng, L.S. (2020, February). Discovery of a novel coronavirus associated with the recent pneumonia outbreak in humans and its potential bat origin.

Nature, 10.1038/s41586-020-2012-7

Zhou, S.J., Wang, G., & Zhang, W.B. (2018). Effect of TLR4/MyD88 signaling pathway on sepsis-associated acute respiratory distress syndrome in rats, via regulation of macrophage activation and inflammatory response. *Experimental and Therapeutic Medicine*, 15(4), 3376–3384. https://doi.org/10.3892/etm.2018.5815

Zhou, Y.X., Li, M., Tang, T.S., Wang, B., & Zhang, B. (2012). A study on Gypsum Compounds and Their Antipyretic Function and Anti-inflammatory Mechanisms. *Journal of Shaanxi College Traditional Chinese Medicine*, 35, 033.

Zhu, Y.P. (1998). *Chinese Materia Medica: Chemistry, Pharmacology and Applications*. CRC Press.

Zielińska, S., & Matkowski, A. (2014). Phytochemistry and bioactivity of aromatic and medicinal plants from the genus Agastache (Lamiaceae). *Phytochemistry Review*, 13(2): 391–416. Apr 3. DOI: 10.1007/s11101-014-9349-1

Zuo, G.Y., Li, Z.Q., Chen, L.R., & Xu, X.J. (2007). Activity of compounds from Chinese herbal medicine Rhodiola kirilowii (Regel), Maxim against hcV nS3 serine protease. *Antiviral Research*, 76:86-92.

More books by Anne Angelone

<u>Functional Scalp Acupuncture</u>

<u>The Acupuncture Trip</u>

<u>The Autoimmune Diet</u>

<u>If The Buddha Had an Autoimmune Disease</u>

<u>The Autoimmune Paleo Breakthrough</u>

<u>The Paleo Autoimmune Protocol</u>

<u>The Histamine Free Paleo Breakthrough</u>

<u>The FODMAP Free Paleo Breakthrough</u>

<u>Gut Clear</u>

<u>Beyond Cannabis</u>

www.ingramcontent.com/pod-product-compliance
Lightning Source LLC
Chambersburg PA
CBHW060414220526
45465CB00008B/2881